May 1995

WITH COMPLIMENTS

acuson

A Colour Atlas of Doppler Ultrasonography in Obstetrics

An Introduction to its Use in Maternal Fetal Medicine

Edited by

KEVIN HARRINGTON MRCPI, MRCOG
and
STUART CAMPBELL FRCOG
*Department of Obstetrics and Gynaecology,
King's College School of Medicine and
Dentistry, London*

Edward Arnold
A member of the Hodder Headline Group
LONDON   BOSTON   MELBOURNE   AUCKLAND

First published in Great Britain 1995
by Edward Arnold, a division of Hodder Headline PLC
338 Euston Road, London NW1 3BH

Distributed in the Americas by
Little, Brown and Company
34 Beacon Street, Boston, MA 02108

Whilst the advice and information in this book is believed to be true and
accurate at the date of going to press, neither the authors nor the publisher
can accept any legal responsibility or liability for any errors or omissions that
may be made. In particular (but without limiting the generality of the
preceding disclaimer) every effort has been made to check drug dosages;
however, it is still possible that errors have been missed. Furthermore,
dosage schedules are constantly being revised and new side-effects
recognized. For these reasons the reader is strongly urged to consult the
drug companies' printed instructions before administering any of the drugs
recommended in this book.

British Library Cataloguing in Publication Data
A catalogue record for this book is available from the British Library

ISBN 0 340 56952 2

1   2   3   4   5   95   96   97   98   99

Typeset in 11/12 Bembo by Wordperfect, Isleworth.
Printed and bound by Dah Hua Printing Press Co. Ltd., Hong Kong.

Contents

Contributors

Stuart Campbell FRCOG
Department of Obstetrics and Gynaecology, King's
    College School of Medicine and Dentistry,
    London

R. G. Carpenter PhD
Department of Medical Statistics, London School of
    Hygiene and Tropical Medicine, London

Colin Deane PhD
Department of Medical Engineering and Physics,
    King's College School of Medicine and Dentistry,
    London

Laurent Fermont MD
Institut de Puériculture de Paris, Paris

Kevin Harrington MRCPI, MRCOG
Department of Obstetrics and Gynaecology, King's
    College School of Medicine and Dentistry,
    London

Kurt Hecher MD
Department of Prenatal Diagnosis and,
    Therapy, AKH Barmleek, Hamburg

Eric Jauniaux MD, PhD
Department of Obstetrics and Gynaecology,
    Academic Hospital Erasme, Free University of
    Brussels (ULB), Brussels

Jérôme Le Bidois MD
Institut de Puériculture de Paris, Paris

Bruce Ramsay MRCOG
Department of Obstetrics and Gynaecology, Chelsea
    and Westminster Hospital, London

Ian Sullivan BMedSc, FRAP
Department of Cardiology, The Hospital for Sick
    Children, London

Preface

Although the clinical use of Doppler ultrasound was first proposed some 35 years ago, it is only in the last decade that its potential in obstetrics has begun to be realized. The advances in ultrasound and computer technology in recent years have enabled the production of ever more sophisticated scanning machines. One of the most exciting of these developments has been the incorporation of colour Doppler imaging (CDI) technology into B-mode/pulsed Doppler duplex scanning machines. With the aid of colour Doppler imaging it is possible to identify, and with pulsed Doppler indirectly quantify, blood flow in vessels and organs that was difficult, if not impossible, to observe before.

CDI allows us to monitor the complex vasculature of the uterus, placenta and fetus during pregnancy. It can be used in the early diagnosis of a wide range of materno-fetal complications and diseases. Because of the potential for colour Doppler applications it seemed prudent to produce a colour atlas to act as an introduction to the technique and its potential when applied to obstetrics. The book commences with a chapter on the physics of Doppler ultrasound. This is an uncomplicated introduction to the world of physics, designed to help those unfamiliar with Doppler to become accustomed to its principles as applied to ultrasound. Chapter 2 attempts to help the beginner overcome the common problems encountered when starting to use colour Doppler ultrasound.

Chapter 3 describes the changes seen in the uterine and fetal circulation in the first trimester. Changes in the uterine circulation in pregnancy are explored in greater detail in Chapter 4, where the transvaginal and transabdominal approach for obtaining signals from the uterine circulation are described. The potential for using uterine Doppler studies as a screening test for the early prediction of uteroplacental complications is discussed. The placenta and umbilical cord are the lifeline of the growing fetus. Chapter 5 demonstrates the role CDI plays in recognizing problems within the placenta and cord. As we do not use CDI for the detection of fetal structural anomalies (other than the fetal heart) on a routine basis, a chapter was not dedicated to this subject.

Chapters 6 and 7 illustrate the technique for obtaining reliable measurements from the fetal arterial and venous circulation and the changes that occur within the vascular system during pregnancy. It is important to appreciate the variation in blood flow within the normal fetus, and the pitfalls when acquiring such Doppler information, so that interpretation of flow velocity waveforms is appropriate Chapter 8 describes the fetal response to hypoxia and anaemia, as seen with the aid of colour Doppler imaging. Doppler studies of the fetal circulation provide information that is often unobtainable from conventional methods of fetal assessment. Therefore, it complements the information deri- ved from other ultrasound techniques, and can be of use in the management of the at risk fetus.

Although the majority of structural cardiac anomalies can be detected with B-mode ultrasound, CDI adds a whole new dimension to fetal echocardiography. Chapter 9 provides a portrait of the changes seen in the structurally normal heart in normal and complicated pregnancies. When a structural lesion is diagnosed it is important to know the likely repercussions for the child, not just after birth, but for the remainder of its life. Many cardiac lesions are straightforward and the prognosis clear. Chapter 10 illustrates the important role Doppler has to play in evaluating complex or rare cardiac anomalies. The information derived about the haemodynamic consequences of cardiac lesions can help in counselling parents and planning future surgery.

Ultrasound technology continues to develop in leaps and bounds. Chapter 11 provides a glimpse of new innovative techniques that are now available for evaluation. As with Doppler ultrasound, it may be some time before we appreciate the role these new advances have to play in our practice.

Producing a chapter for a colour atlas requires an author to write a text that is informative yet easy to follow and, more importantly, to strive to produce a collection of images that clearly illustrate the particular point being made. We are grateful to all the authors in this book, for the time and effort they have employed in producing chapters that are easy to read and that contain images of the highest standard.

We trust that this atlas will be of interest to all those involved in the care of the pregnant woman, and in particular people who perform obstetric ultrasound. A colour atlas cannot by itself produce a competent and skilled operator: this process is dependent on good, practical training and a dedicated approach on the part of the sonographer. With the aid of a well-illustrated atlas the process of becoming capable at performing and interpreting Doppler information will be made a little more enjoyable, interesting and exciting. That is the aim of this atlas. We hope that it achieves this objective for you.

KH and SC

Doppler ultrasound: physical principles

Colin Deane

INTRODUCTION

Doppler ultrasound is now a widely used technique for the investigation of blood flow. A large range of equipment is available from inexpensive hand-held devices providing an audio interpretation of blood movement to sophisticated colour flow scanners in which a colour map of moving flow signals is superimposed on a B-mode image to provide a dynamic interpretation of flow phenomena.

As equipment has developed, so has the range of applications and the confidence in the information obtained. The attractions for the clinician are several: Doppler ultrasound is non-invasive, it provides real-time information and the equipment can usually be moved to the patient when necessary.

With such versatility, it is tempting to employ the technique for ever more demanding applications and to try to measure increasingly subtle changes in the circulation within vascular beds. To avoid misinterpretation of results, however, it is essential for the user of Doppler ultrasound to be aware of the factors which affect the Doppler signal, be it a colour Doppler image (CDI) or a Doppler sonogram. Competent use of Doppler ultrasound techniques requires an understanding of three key components:

- haemodynamics within vessels;
- the capabilities and limitations of Doppler ultrasound;
- the different parameters which contribute to the Doppler sonogram.

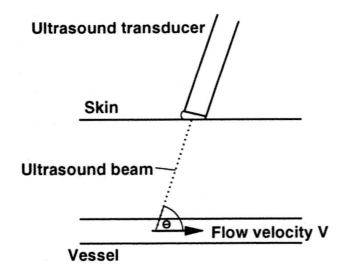

Fig. 1.1
The origin of the Doppler signal. The ultrasound transducer transmits ultrasound in the direction of the beam. The movement of red blood cells imparts frequency shifts in the reflection back to the transducer dependent on the velocity of blood flow and beam/flow angle Θ (equation 1).

The aim of this chapter is to describe the principles of Doppler ultrasound and to show how these components contribute to Doppler ultrasound images such as those presented in this book. Common pitfalls which can give rise to ambiguous or poor quality images will be described. Chapter 2 will illustrate how to set up Doppler ultrasound equipment to obtain good images. For further reading in the subject there are texts available covering Doppler ultrasound and blood flow theory in detail.[1, 2]

Blood flow is a dynamic process; the beauty of Doppler ultrasound is that it provides dynamic images of flow phenomena. The images shown here are, of necessity, static ones. Where applicable, multiple images are presented to illustrate changes over time. In the end, however, there is no substitution for seeing Doppler ultrasound practised 'live' when its full capabilities may be shown to best advantage.

THE DOPPLER PRINCIPLE APPLIED TO ULTRASOUND

In medical imaging, the term Doppler ultrasound encompasses continuous wave Doppler (CW), pulsed wave Doppler (PW) and colour Doppler imaging (CDI). Processing for each differs considerably but the underlying principles are similar. When ultrasound is reflected from a moving target, in this case red blood cells, the movement of the target causes a frequency shift in the reflected signal. This frequency shift is detected by the ultrasound receiver.

The frequency shift f_d, known as the Doppler shift frequency or Doppler frequency, can be related to the flow velocity v (Fig. 1.1) within a vessel by the Doppler equation which approximates as follows:

$$f_d = \frac{2 f_t v \cos \theta}{c} \qquad \text{(Eq. 1)}$$

where f_t is the transmitted ultrasound frequency, c is the velocity of sound in tissue and θ is the angle between the ultrasound beam and the direction of flow. (Flow velocity is normally assumed to be along the axis of the vessel and θ is often described as the beam/vessel angle. This assumption is not always true.)

Since changes in c for different tissue types are relatively small, the Doppler frequency is substantially altered by three factors:

1 The magnitude of the Doppler frequency increases as blood flow **velocity** (v) increases.
2 The Doppler frequency increases as the transmitted ultrasound **frequency** (f_t) increases. This means that higher frequency probes are more sensitive to low flow velocities. Unfortunately, attenuation of ultra-

sound in tissue is frequency dependent so that high frequency probes (5 MHz and above) may not provide adequate penetration when examining deep vessels.Conversely, the use of low frequency ultrasound in deep abdominal vessels may lead to low flow velocities not being detected.

3 The Doppler frequency increases as the Doppler ultrasound beam becomes more aligned to the flow direction (θ becomes smaller). This is of the utmost importance in the use of Doppler ultrasound. The implications are illustrated schematically in Fig. 1.2.

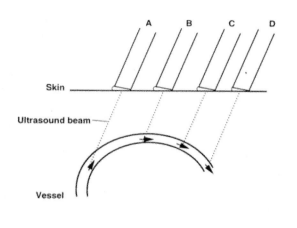

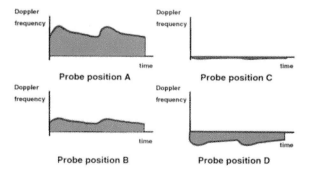

Fig. 1.2
The effect of the beam/flow angle on the Doppler frequency shift. The diagram shows a curved vessel of constant diameter and velocity. Representative Doppler frequency sonograms for an arterial-type flow are shown below. At probe position A the beam is nearly aligned with the vessel. Flow is towards the beam and produces positive Doppler shift frequencies. Doppler frequencies are greater than they are for probe position B, where the angle is approximately 65°. At probe position C the beam/flow angle is close to 90° resulting in very low Doppler frequencies. At probe position D the flow is away from the beam; Doppler shift frequencies are negative.

All Doppler ultrasound equipment employs filters to cut out the high amplitude, low frequency Doppler signals resulting from tissue movement, for instance due to vessel wall motion. In some machines this threshold can be altered to cut out frequencies below, for ex-

ample, 50, 100 or 200 Hz. This filter frequency limits the minimum flow velocities that can be measured, the actual value being dependent on the transmitted frequency and beam/flow angle.

CONTINUOUS WAVE DOPPLER ULTRASOUND

Continuous wave (CW) ultrasound is the simplest type of Doppler ultrasound. Because CW systems transmit and receive ultrasound continuously, Doppler shifts are obtained from all vessels in the path of the ultrasound beam (until the ultrasound becomes sufficiently attenuated due to depth). Although CW systems are not range specific, they do have some advantages over pulsed wave (PW) systems, most notably in that they do not have an upper limit to the Doppler shift which can be measured.

The received Doppler shifted signal is processed to isolate the Doppler frequency shift (*fd* in equation 1). The Doppler frequency can be amplified to produce an audio signal. (Practical transmitted frequencies and blood velocities produce Doppler shifts in the audio range.) Further signal processing can provide directional information (whether the flow is towards the probe or away from it) or an analysis of the range of frequency shifts occurring (the spectral display, also known as the sonogram) (Fig. 1.3).

Relatively inexpensive Doppler ultrasound systems are available which employ CW probes to give Doppler output without the addition of B-mode images. One disadvantage of a Doppler only system is that the

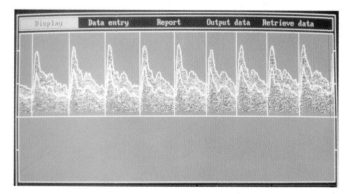

Fig. 1.3
The Doppler sonogram. The graphical representation of the Doppler shift frequencies shows time on the horizontal axis and frequency shift along the vertical axis. At every point in time there is a range of frequencies because of the range of velocities through the vessel cross-section. The amplitude of the frequencies is represented by different colours (yellow – high, red – low). The maximum and mean frequencies of the sonogram have been calculated and are shown as white lines. There is a region close to the x-axis in which no spectrum is shown due to the high-pass filter.

beam/flow angle θ may not be known, preventing velocity measurements being derived from the Doppler frequency shifts.

PULSED WAVE DOPPLER ULTRASOUND

A limitation of CW systems is that they are not range specific, which can make it difficult to isolate the Doppler signals from a particular vessel. Pulsed wave (PW) systems transmit short pulses of ultrasound, the echoes of which are received after a short interval of time. PW systems allow measurement of the depth (or

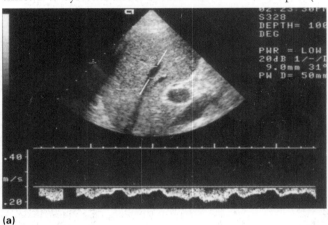

(a)

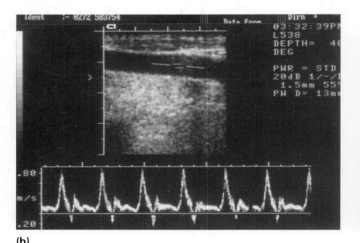

(b)

Fig. 1.4 *Pulsed Doppler in a duplex scanner.*
(a) Phased array (sector) transducer. The sample volume (gate) is set to insonate the entire cross-section of the vein. Flow is away from the transducer and produces negative frequency shifts. A beam/flow angle correction is made and velocities are measured. (b) Linear array transducer. Flow is from right to left. The Doppler beam is steered to the right to give a beam/flow angle of 55°. The Doppler sample volume is 1.5 mm in length, placed in the middle of the artery to measure the high flow velocities in the centre. Flow towards the beam produces positive frequency shifts. A beam/flow angle correction is made to calculate flow velocities.

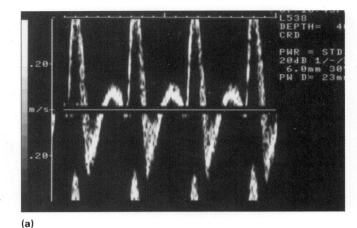

(a)

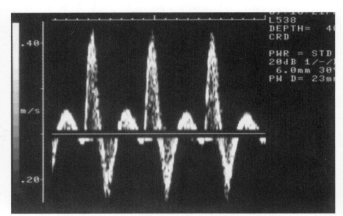

(b)

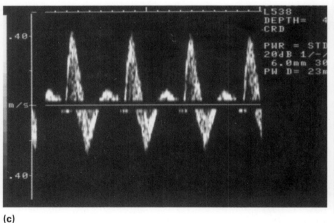

(c)

Fig. 1.5 *Aliasing in pulsed Doppler and methods for correcting it.*
(a) The sonogram is ambiguous with peak systolic signals exceeding the maximum scale on the y-axis. The high Doppler frequency shifts are misinterpreted as negative shifts because the pulse repetition frequency is not sufficiently high. (b) By changing the baseline, the positive frequency/velocity scale is extended at the expense of the negative scale. The flow waveform is now shown unambiguously. (c) An alternative to changing the baseline. Increasing the pulse repetition frequency (PRF) changes the y-axis velocity scale. The flow waveform is interpreted clearly.

range) at which blood flow is observed (by measurement of the time taken for the pulse to be transmitted to and reflected back from the blood cells). Additionally, the size of the sample volume (or range gate) can be changed by altering the transmitted pulse length and the time over which the signal is received. In this way, the region of examination of blood flow can be altered to suit the specific clinical requirement (Fig. 1.4).

Aliasing

PW systems suffer from a practical limitation. When pulses are transmitted at a given sampling frequency (known as the pulse repetition frequency, PRF), the maximum Doppler frequency shift fd that can be measured unambiguously is half the PRF. If the blood velocity and beam/flow angle being measured combine to give a fd value greater than half of the PRF, ambiguity of the Doppler shift occurs. This ambiguity is known as aliasing (Fig. 1.5). (A common analogy is that of wagon wheels in films which can appear to be going backwards due to the low frame rate of film causing misinterpretation of the movement of the wheel spokes.)

The PRF is itself constrained by the range of the sample volume. The time interval between sampling pulses must be sufficient for a pulse to make the return journey from transducer to the reflector and back. If a second pulse is sent before the first is received, the receiver cannot discriminate between the reflected signal from both pulses and ambiguity of the range of the sample volume ensues. As depth of investigation increases, the journey time of the pulse to and from the reflector is increased, reducing the PRF for unambiguous ranging. The result is that the maximum fd measurable decreases with depth.

Some manufacturers offer a facility whereby range ambiguity is permitted, allowing high PRFs to be used to measure high Doppler shifts. This results in one or more additional range gates being sampled.

DUPLEX DOPPLER ULTRASOUND

Duplex ultrasound (also referred to as image directed Doppler ultrasound) scanners combine Doppler and B-mode ultrasound. The advantages are that the B-mode image can be used to guide the Doppler beam and that blood flow information can be combined with anatomical and structural information. If the course of the vessel being examined is evident, correction for the Doppler beam/flow angle θ may be made, permitting an estimate of flow velocity.

Most duplex ultrasound scanners currently available allow simultaneous real-time Doppler and B-mode imaging (often at different frequencies to optimize both modes). The Doppler beam can be steered and, if PW

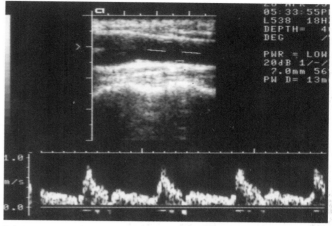

(a)

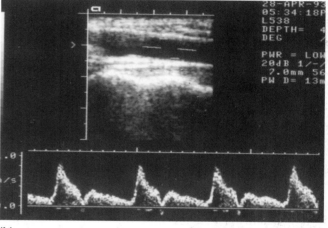

(b)

Fig. 1.6 *Duplex ultrasound.*
(a) B-mode and PW Doppler are used concurrently. The transducer elements are shared between modes. (b) The B-mode is frozen while the PW Doppler is operating. The transducer elements are used solely for PW Doppler. The temporal resolution of the sonogram is improved over that in (a).

Doppler is used, the sample volume can be placed specifically in the region of interest (Fig. 1.4). The temporal resolution of the sonogram may be improved by freezing the image and using the transducer elements solely for the Doppler mode (Fig. 1.6).

COLOUR DOPPLER IMAGING (CDI)

Colour Doppler imaging (CDI) – also referred to as Doppler flow imaging (CFI) or colour Doppler ultrasound (CDU) – produces a colour coded map of Doppler frequency shifts superimposed onto a B-mode ultrasound image. Although CDI uses PW ultrasound, its processing differs from that used to provide the

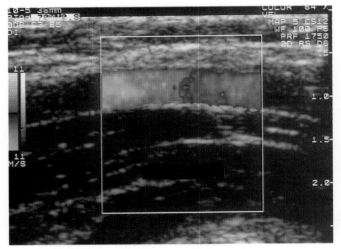

(a)

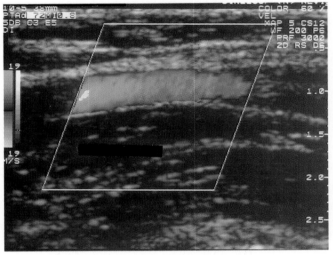

(b)

Fig. 1.7 *Colour Doppler imaging, effect of beam/flow angle – linear array.*
(a) The colour is assigned as red for flow towards the ultrasound beam (positive frequency shift), blue away from it. Flow in the vessel is from left to right. The direction of the beam is perpendicular to the transducer. The vessel lies nearly parallel to the skin surface. In the left half of the image, there is a velocity component towards the beam producing positive shifts (red). In the left half of the image, there is a velocity component away from the beam as the vessel goes deeper. Frequency shifts are negative (blue). (b) The direction of the beam has been electronically steered to provide a better beam/flow angle. The colour assignment is now blue for flow towards the beam (positive frequency shifts). Flow is from left to right and has a velocity component towards the beam throughout its length. Flow appears as blue. To the left of the image, lighter shades of blue show increased frequency shifts where the curvature of the vessel produces a lower beam/flow angle.

Doppler sonogram. The latter employs several long pulses to enable a full spectral analysis of the region of interest to be obtained over a small interval of time. This is repeated to generate the sonogram in real time.

Since CDI may have to produce several thousand colour pixels of flow information for each frame superimposed on the B-mode image, analysis is less complex. CDI uses fewer, shorter pulses along each colour scan line of the image to give a mean frequency shift and a variance at each small area of measurement. This frequency shift is converted to a colour pixel. The scanner then repeats this for several lines to build up the colour image which is superimposed onto the B-mode image (Fig. 1.7). The transducer elements are switched rapidly between B-mode and CDI to give an impression of a combined simultaneous image. The pulses used for CDI are typically 3–4 times longer than those for the B-mode image with a corresponding loss of axial resolution.

Colour assignment

Assignment of colour to frequency shifts is usually based on direction (e.g. red for Doppler shifts towards the ultrasound beam and blue for shifts away from it) and magnitude (different colour hues or lighter saturations for higher frequency shifts).[3] Colour assignments can be reversed (compare Figures 1.7a and 1.7b). In most systems, it is possible to highlight a range of Doppler shifts in a contrasting colour (Fig. 1.8).

The colour Doppler image is dependent on general Doppler factors, particularly the need for a good beam/flow angle. Because the beams in a linear array transducer are unidirectional, curved vessels can have different colour hues and possibly colour reversal throughout the area of investigation (Fig. 1.7). Phased array and curvilinear transducers have a radiating pattern of ultrasound beams so that a straight vessel pro-

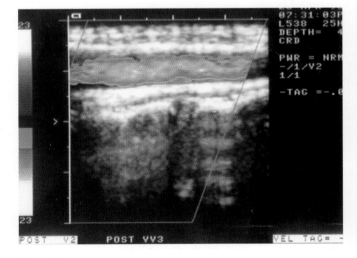

Fig. 1.8
Flow is from right to left. The beam is steered with red assigned for negative frequency shifts. The flow velocity component is away from the beam so appears as red. Green has been used to highlight low frequency shifts resulting from the low flow velocities near the wall.

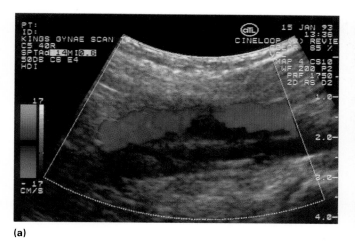

(a)

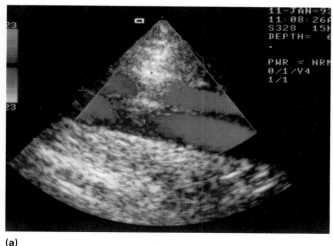

(a)

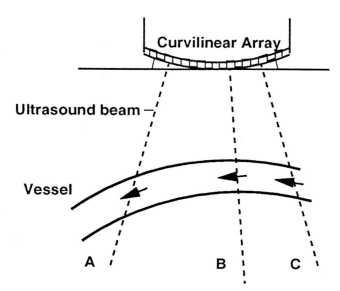

(b)

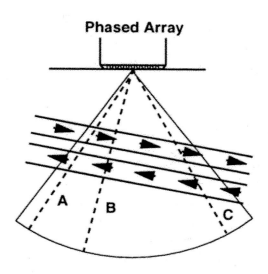

(b)

Fig. 1.9 *Colour Doppler imaging – curvilinear array.*
The colour image (a) shows a vessel with flow from right to left. The colour assignment is red as positive frequency shifts. The diagram (b) shows how the radiating beam pattern produces the colour image. At beam A, flow is away from the beam producing negative frequency shifts (blue). At B, beam/flow angles are nearly 90° producing no frequency shift or colour. At beam C, flow is towards the beam; frequency shift is positive (red).

Fig. 1.10 *Colour Doppler imaging – phased array.*
The colour image (a) shows a phased array (sector) transducer imaging two vessels. Flow in the upper vessel is from left to right and in the lower from right to left. The colour scale is set with blue to represent flow towards the transducer and red away from it. The diagram (b) shows how the colour image arises. Along beam A, the flow in the upper vessel has a velocity vector towards the beam (blue), in the lower vessel the velocity vector is away from the beam (red). Along beam C, the position is reversed. Along beam B both vessels are close to a beam/flow angle of 90°, there is no colour image.

duces variation in colour as the beam/vessel angle changes (Figs 1.9 and 1.10).

As with B-mode ultrasound, the presence of highly attenuating structures (particularly bone) within tissue can lead to a loss of colour image (Fig. 1.11).

Flow sensitivity/filters/flow discrimination

Increased sensitivity to low velocity flow can be achieved by decreasing the pulse repetition rate (some manufacturers call this altering the scale). However, by

reducing PRF, aliasing of the colour image occurs at lower velocities. Aliasing in colour flow appears as colour wrap-around because the colour scale is essentially a circular one. The effect is shown in Fig. 1.12. Flow conditions may arise in a colour flow image in which a colour can represent aliased flow in one direction and reverse flow elsewhere in the image (Fig. 1.13). As in PW Doppler, the maximum PRF is limited

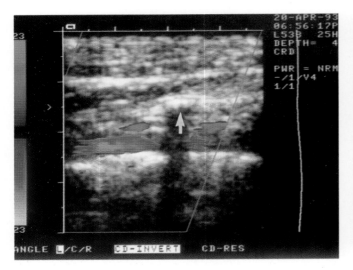

Fig. 1.11
The high attenuation of ultrasound by bone (arrowed) causes a loss of both B-mode and CDI image.

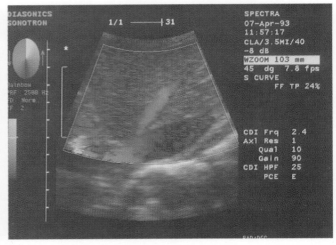

Fig. 1.14
Colour flow signal from tissue. 'Flow' images have been detected both in blood vessels and in tissue due to movement of the probe. This artefact can also occur due to tissue movement (e.g. patient breathing).

by the depth of the investigation. Consequently, the maximum unambiguous frequency shift decreases as the depth of CDI investigation increases.

As previously described, tissue movement can give rise to strong low frequency Doppler signals. Colour Doppler images of blood flow can be obscured by overlaying of colour from this source where there is significant tissue movement (Fig. 1.14). Ultimately, sensitivity to low velocity flow is limited by the filter frequency used to eliminate noise from tissue motion. Manufacturers have gone to considerable effort to develop motion discrimination methods which differentiate signals from tissue movement and blood flow.

If an operator experiences difficulty in registering

low velocity flows, Doppler frequency shifts may be increased by reducing beam/vessel angle or using higher frequency ultrasound. However, there is always a threshold flow velocity below which Doppler ultrasound will not be able to detect flow. *The lack of observable Doppler shifts in a vessel does not necessarily mean that there is no flow in it.*

Frame rate

The use of CDI can decrease the available frame rate, because the same transducer elements are used for both B-mode and CDI. For each frame, B-mode imaging

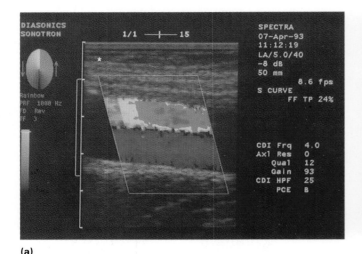

(a)

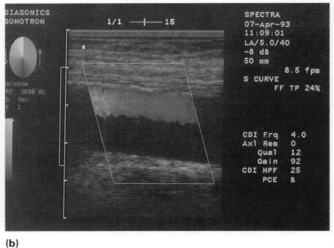

(b)

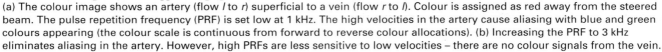

Fig. 1.12 *Aliasing in colour Doppler imaging – I.*
(a) The colour image shows an artery (flow *l* to *r*) superficial to a vein (flow *r* to *l*). Colour is assigned as red away from the steered beam. The pulse repetition frequency (PRF) is set low at 1 kHz. The high velocities in the artery cause aliasing with blue and green colours appearing (the colour scale is continuous from forward to reverse colour allocations). (b) Increasing the PRF to 3 kHz eliminates aliasing in the artery. However, high PRFs are less sensitive to low velocities – there are no colour signals from the vein.

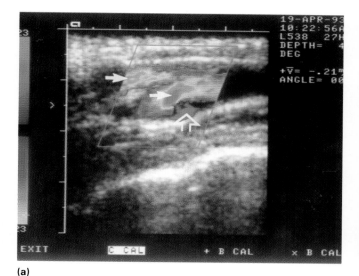

(a)

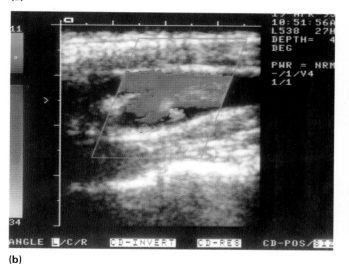

(b)

Fig. 1.13 *Aliasing in colour Doppler imaging – II.*
(a) The flow in the Arteryis from right to left. The colour beams are steered with red away from the beam (negative frequency shift). The colour image shows regions of aliased flow (solid arrows) where high velocities result in frequencies exceeding the maximum of the negative range. The image shows a region of flow in which the velocity vector is towards the beam (open arrow). (This is sometimes referred to as reverse flow – strictly it is reversed in the direction of the colour beam, not of the vessel.) (b) By extending the range of negative frequency shift colour assignment (red) and reducing the positive shift range (blue), the aliasing is eliminated. (This is often referred to as altering the colour baseline.)

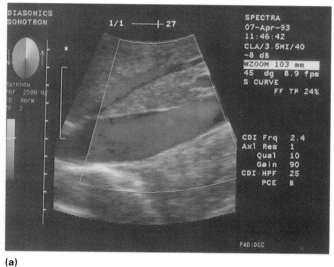

(a)

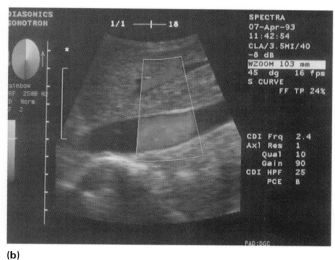

(b)

Fig. 1.15 *Effect of CDI on frame rate.*
(a) The area of CDI investigation is large, requiring a correspondingly large number of scan lines. Frame rate is 8.9 frames per second (fps). (b) The area of CDI has been reduced. Fewer scan lines are required to produce each image frame. Frame rate rises to 16 fps.

requires only one pulse per scan line, CDI typically requires 5–10. Broadly, the frame rate increases with increased pulse repetition frequency, but decreases as the number of colour lines increases (e.g. due to a large area of colour flow examination) and decreases as the number of pulses per line is increased (to improve the quality of the colour signal). The effects and their consequences are summarized in Table 1.1.

The loss of frame rate can be of particular importance in obstetric scanning where the fast fetal heart rate results in rapid changes in instantaneous flow. Since the PRF setting is usually governed by considerations of aliasing and sensitivity to low velocity flow, other factors may be altered to give the optimum frame rate for the examination. The most important of these is the advantage which can be gained by reducing the area of the image under CDI investigation (Fig. 1.15).

Additionally, some manufacturers allow a trade-off between pixel size and frame rate by reducing the line density (Fig. 1.16) and hence spatial resolution. In some scanners, the operator can vary the number of pulses per scan line to trade quality of image for frame rate (Fig. 1.17). Manufacturers may also offer control of

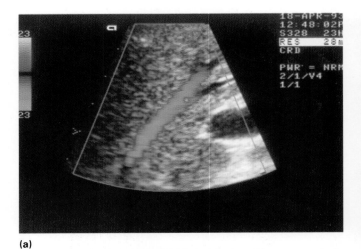

(a)

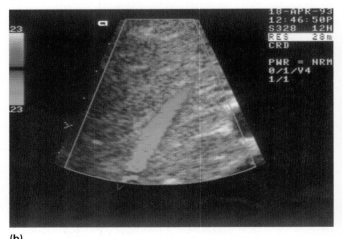

(b)

Fig. 1.16 *Effect of scan line density on frame rate.*
(a) The image is of a small region of tissue showing vessel detail. Frame rate is 23 fps; the edges of the colour image of the flow appear ragged because of the low scan line density. (b) The scan line density is increased. The need for more scan lines reduces frame rate to 12 fps. The edges of the colour image of flow appear to have smoother edges.

colour image persistence, where information from previous frames of colour flow are added to the most recent frame. This can be helpful in identifying transient low flow velocities but can give a false impression of the flow dynamics. Although these facilities exist, they are often not employed extensively in day-to-day scanning. Manufacturers give guidelines as to the best set-up of these controls for specific applications; they are usually set up at the press of an application/examination/set-up key.

Focusing

In duplex ultrasound scanners, PW Doppler is automatically focused to obtain the best signal from the area under investigation. With CDI, the area of investigation may be large. The focus zone of the image should be

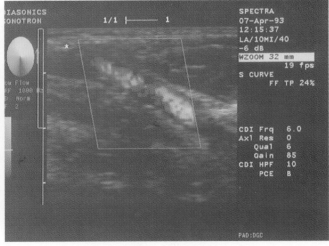

(a)

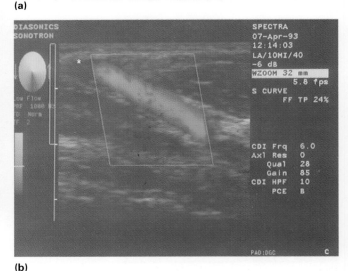

(b)

Fig. 1.17 *Effect of colour 'quality' on frame rate.*
(a) The frame rate is 19 fps. The colour image of the vessel is incomplete, although it is sufficient for most diagnostic purposes. (b) By changing the 'quality' setting, the number of pulses sent on each scan line is increased, improving the frequency shift information and thus the colour appearance of the vessel. Frame rate falls to 5.8 fps.

placed adjacent to the region of specific interest to obtain the best CDI image there.

Colour velocity imaging (CVI)

Recently, one manufacturer has introduced a colour flow imaging mode known as colour velocity imaging (CVI). In colour Doppler scanners, the change in phase shift between the received pulse echoes is used to reconstruct the Doppler shift. In CVI, the change in the time between transmission and reception of pulse echoes in consecutive pulses is used to calculate the distance travelled between pulses. Like CDI, this gives a velocity vector in the direction of the scan line which is converted into a colour pixel. The processing of each

Table 1.1 Factors affecting colour flow image and frame rate.

	Advantages	*Disadvantages*
Increased PRF	Aliasing occurs at high Doppler frequencies Can improve frame rate	Less sensitive to low flow velocities
Decreased PRF	Improved sensitivity to low flow velocities	Aliasing occurs at low Doppler frequencies Frame rate may decrease
Increased number of colour scan lines	Used to increase area of colour imaging *or* Line density can be increased to give better resolution of the colour image	Frame rate falls as more colour scan lines are used
Increased number of pulses per scan line	Quality of information is enhanced with improved colour definition	Frame rate falls because of the need for more pulses per image

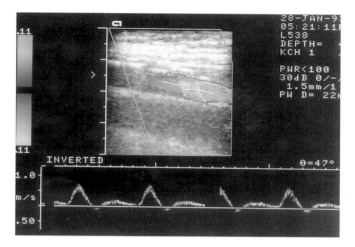

Fig. 1.19
CDI with spectral PW Doppler sonogram of an artery (flow *l* to *r*). The B-mode/CDI are updated every 3 seconds. During updating, the PW Doppler is switched off (note the gap in the sonogram at the end of the second cardiac cycle, which lasts until peak systole in the third). The colour scan is built up from left to right of the colour box in this interval. The colour changes from none at the left of the box (end diastolic flow) to red, then yellow, then blue (aliased) as the flow velocity accelerates in systole.

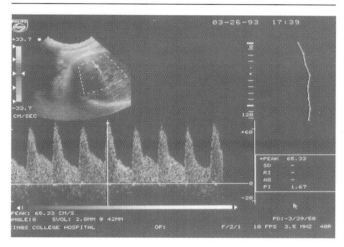

Fig. 1.18
The colour flow image shows the course of the middle cerebral artery and enables an angle corrected pulsed Doppler cursor to be placed accurately.

mode is described elsewhere.[4] Among the stated advantages of CVI are that aliasing does not occur (although there are other velocity range limits arising from the signal processing) and that the use of shorter B-mode-like pulses gives improved axial resolution (see Chapter 11). As with CDI, use of CVI decreases the B-mode frame rate.

Colour Doppler imaging with 'spectral' Doppler

Since CDI (and CVI) provides a limited amount of information over a large region and spectral Doppler

provides a lot of information about a small region, the two modes are complementary and in practice should be used as such. Although CDI machines can be provided with both CW and PW Doppler, for work in obstetrics and gynaecology, PW Doppler is most likely to be used.

CDI can be used to identify vessels to be examined, to identify the presence and direction of flow, to highlight gross circulation anomalies throughout the entire CDI image and to provide beam/vessel angle correction for velocity measurements. PW Doppler is used to provide analysis of the flow at specific sites in the vessel under investigation (Fig. 1.18).

When using CDI with PW Doppler, the CDI/B-mode image is frozen while the PW Doppler is activated. (Recently, some manufacturers have produced concurrent CDI and PW Doppler but with reduced performance of each mode – see below.) The CDI mode may be set to update whereby at a pre-set interval the PW Doppler ceases for a short interval while the transducer elements and circuitry are devoted to producing a CDI/B-mode image. The colour image may show a range of colour assignments in the vessel due to change in flow in the time taken to produce the image (Fig. 1.19).

Simultaneous colour Doppler imaging/spectral Doppler

Some manufacturers now offer facilities whereby simultaneous real-time colour Doppler imaging and spectral

Doppler can be employed. This is sometimes referred to as triplex scanning. When these modes are used simultaneously, performance of each is decreased. Because transducer elements are employed in three modes (B-mode, colour flow and PW Doppler), frame rate is lowered and the available PRF range may be reduced.

BLOOD FLOW MEASUREMENTS USING DOPPLER ULTRASOUND

Velocity measurement

Theoretically, once the beam/flow angle is known, velocities can be calculated from the Doppler spectrum as shown in the Doppler equation. However, errors in the measured velocity may still occur.[1,5] Sources of error can be broadly divided into three categories.

1 Errors can arise in the formation of the Doppler spectrum due to:

- use of multiple elements in array transducers;
- non-uniform insonation of the vessel lumen;
- insonation of more than one vessel;
- use of filters removing low velocity components;
- intrinsic spectral broadening (reflectors passing through a beam produce a range of Doppler shifts because of the geometry of the transmitted beam and the reflected ultrasound).[1]

2 Errors can arise in the measurement of the ultrasound beam/flow velocity angle. Use of high angles ($\theta > 60°$) may give rise to error because of the comparatively large changes in cosine which occur with small changes of angle. Additionally, the velocity vector may not be in the direction of the vessel axis.

3 Errors can arise in the calculation packages which the manufacturers provide for analysis of the Doppler spectrum (for instance, of intensity weighted mean velocity).

While efforts can be made to minimize errors, the operator should be aware of their likely range. It is good practice to try to repeat velocity measurements, if possible using a different beam approach, to gain a feel for the variability of measurements in a particular application. However, even repeated measurements may not reveal systematic errors occurring in a particular machine.

The effort to produce accurate velocity measurements should be balanced against the importance of absolute velocity measurements for an investigation. Changes in velocity (such as occur through a stenosis) are often of more clinical relevance when making a

diagnosis. In this and other cases, absolute values of velocity measurement may not be required.

Calculation of absolute flow

Total flow measurement using colour or duplex Doppler ultrasound is fraught with difficulties, even under ideal conditions.[5, 6] Errors which may arise include:

- inaccurate measurement of vessel cross-sectional area (arteries pulsate during the cardiac cycle);
- errors in the derivation of velocity (see above).

These errors become particularly large when flow calculations are made in small vessels; errors in measurement of diameter are magnified when used to derive cross-sectional area. As with velocity measurements, it is prudent to be aware of possible errors and to conduct repeatability tests.

Flow waveform analysis

Non-dimensional analysis of the flow waveform shape and spectrum has proved to be a useful technique in the investigation of many vascular beds. It has the advantage that derived indices are independent of the beam/flow angle θ.

The flow waveform shape arises from the action of a pulsatile pressure waveform acting on a distal impedance. Changes in flow waveform shape have been used to investigate both proximal disease (e.g. in the adult peripheral arterial circulation) and distal changes in fetal circulations). While the breadth of uses shows the technique to be versatile, it also serves as a reminder of the range of factors which cause changes to the local Doppler spectrum. If waveform analysis is to be used to observe changes in one component of the proximal or distal vasculature, consideration must be made to ensure that other components are not affecting the waveform significantly.

FLOW WAVEFORM SHAPE – INDICES OF MEASUREMENT

It is beyond the scope of this chapter to detail the various indices which have been used to describe the shape of flow waveforms. Techniques range from simple indices of systolic to diastolic flow to feature extraction methods such as principal component analysis. All are designed to describe the waveform in a quantitative way, usually as a guide to some kind of classification. In general they are a compromise between simplicity and the amount of information obtained. The most common techniques are described more fully elsewhere with discussion of their advantages and disadvantages.[1, 2, 7a, 7b]

The following indices are described briefly because they are commonly used in many vascular beds and because the calculations necessary to produce them are available on many commercial ultrasound scanners. They are all based on the maximum Doppler shift waveform. The heights referred to are of the outline of the waveform (Fig. 1.20) which can be in units of frequency or velocity; all indices are non-dimensional.

POURCELOT'S RESISTANCE INDEX

Pourcelot's resistance index (RI),[8] also known as the resistance index or resistive index, is defined as;

$$RI = \frac{\text{Peak systolic height} - \text{Minimum diastolic height}}{\text{Peak systolic height}}$$

$$RI = \frac{S - D}{S} \qquad \text{(Eq. 2)}$$

As diastolic flow falls, the value of the RI increases; if there is no diastolic flow, the $RI = 1$. RI values greater than 1 are possible if there is reversed diastolic flow.

SYSTOLIC/DIASTOLIC RATIO (AB RATIO)

The systolic/diastolic ratio (S/D, Fig. 1.20) is calculated by dividing the peak systolic height by the minimum diastolic height. As diastolic flow falls, S/D increases; when there is no diastolic flow, the S/D ratio is infinity. In obstetrics, this index is also referred to as the A/B or AB ratio.

PULSATILITY INDEX

Pulsatility index (PI)[9] is defined as:

$$PI = \frac{\text{Peak systolic height} - \text{Minimum diastolic height}}{\text{Mean waveform height}}$$

$$PI = \frac{S - D}{M} \qquad \text{(Eq. 3)}$$

Because of the need to measure the mean height of the waveform, this takes slightly longer to calculate than RI or the S/D ratio. It does, however, give a broader range of values, for instance in describing a range of waveform shapes when there is no end diastolic flow.

In addition to these indices, the flow waveform may be described or categorized by the presence or absence of a particular feature. Two examples are shown in Fig. 1.21: the absence of end diastolic flow and the presence of a post-systolic notch.

Generally, a low pulsatility waveform is indicative of low distal resistance and high pulsatility waveforms occur in high resistance vascular beds (Fig. 1.21),

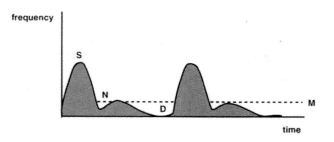

Fig. 1.20
Diagrammatic representation of a flow waveform. S is peak systolic velocity, D is minimum diastolic velocity and M is the mean height of the waveform. There is a post-systolic notch (N) and no flow at end diastole.

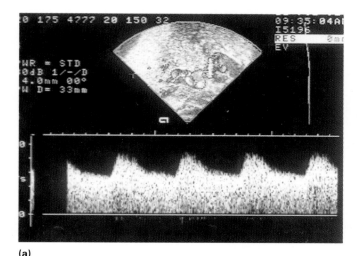

(a)

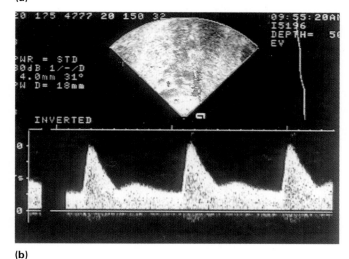

(b)

Fig. 1.21
(a) The flow waveform of a uterine artery shows high diastolic flow. Index measurements are RI = 0.3, PI = 0.45, AB ratio 1.4.
(b) The contralateral uterine artery shows less diastolic flow, a more pulsatile appearance and a post-systolic notch, indicating raised distal resistance. Index measurements are RI - 0.7, PI = 1.45, AB ratio 3.3.

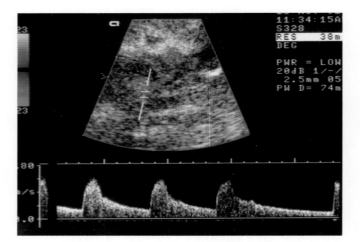

Fig. 1.22
The sonogram shows an arterial flow waveform in a patient with an irregular heart rate. Pulsatility index in the first two cardiac cycles is 1.4 and in the third is 2.3. The example is an extreme one but it illustrates the change in calculated parameters that can arise due to altered heart rate.

although the presence of proximal stenosis, vascular steal or arteriovenous fistulas can modify waveform shape. Care should be taken when trying to interpret indices as an absolute measurement of either upstream or downstream factors. For example, alterations in heart rate can alter the flow waveform shape in a vessel and cause significant changes in the value of indices (Fig. 1.22).

SAFETY

Ultrasound is generally converted into heat energy as it is absorbed by tissue. The heat is lost through conduction and perfusion. To date there have been no harmful effects reported due to the use of diagnostic ultrasound in humans. However, the output power of ultrasound in PW Doppler and colour Doppler modes is many times that of B-mode imaging and there has been concern at the power output available in some currently used diagnostic ultrasound scanners which approaches power levels previously used therapeutically. In obstetric practice, it has been noted that the use of transvaginal probes brings the power source (the transducer head) closer to the embryo and fetus than abdominal transducers, possibly increasing the delivery of energy to the embryo/fetus.

In response to these concerns, the World Federation for Ultrasound in Medicine and Biology (WFUMB) sponsored a series of meetings of experts in the field of ultrasonics and thermal bioeffects. This culminated in statements and recommendations concerning safety of the thermal effects of diagnostic ultrasound examinations.[10] In reviewing the evidence on the adverse effect of heat on tissue (including embryonic tissue), they

recommended that diagnostic exposures that produce a maximum temperature rise of 1.5°C above normal physiological levels may be used without reservation in clinical examination.

Measurement of the actual temperature rise due to an ultrasound investigation is difficult. Because of the problems in measuring intensity *in vivo, in vitro* measurements are made and corrections made for tissues. The accuracy of the calculated *in vivo* measurement is dependent on that of the model. Furthermore, it is difficult to calculate an increase in tissue temperature arising from an estimated intensity. Temperature rise is highly dependent on tissue structure and perfusion.

The US Food and Drug Administration (FDA) have produced guidelines as to the maximum *in situ* value of ultrasound intensity to be used in different clinical applications. The maximum value recommended for fetal work is SPTA (spatial peak temporal average) of 94 mWcm^{-2}. Manufacturers offer a range of user-selected transmitted power levels for all modes of scanning and produce guidelines for use in obstetrics applications. It should be noted that some modern equipment is capable of producing SPTA values of >500 mWcm^{-2} in colour and Doppler modes, which exceeds the FDA guidelines.

The energy delivered to a region of tissue is a product of the power output and the time of investigation (the exposure time). In order to minimize delivery of ultrasound energy to the patient, the following practices should be employed when conducting a scan.

1 Start with the B-mode image (which has the lowest power output) and progress the investigation to include colour flow and Doppler modes. When CDI and Doppler modes are not required, switch them off.
2 Set transmitted power levels to the lowest level which will give an adequate signal (especially in CDI and Doppler modes). Do not exceed the manufacturer's guidelines for the particular application.
3 Do not scan for longer than is necessary to complete the examination.

Transducer surface heating

It has been reported[11] that heating of a transducer surface can occur if the transducer is left transmitting when not in use. The authors observed that in one case, a transducer left operating in air in PW Doppler mode produced a temperature *rise* on its surface of more than 50°C which could cause patient discomfort when applied to the skin. While it is unlikely that this would occur in competent scanning, it is generally good practice to stop transmission of ultrasound (for example, by freezing the image) when the transducer is not in use.

Summary

This chapter has outlined the principles of Doppler ultrasound as they apply to commercial scanners now available. The advantages and limitations of CW, PW and colour flow modes have been described. The physics and instrumentation that contribute to the creation of the Doppler image have been presented together with illustrations as to how the Doppler image can be altered by adjusting mode and scanning parameters. Measurement techniques commonly used to describe Doppler signals have been summarized and a brief introduction to safety considerations has been given. In the following chapter, a step-by-step guide will show how to obtain the optimum Doppler image in each mode in order to use the technique to best advantage.

Acknowledgements

The author is grateful to staff of Diasonics Sonotron, ATL, Acuson and SciMed and to colleagues within King's College Hospital for their help in obtaining some of the images used in this chapter.

References

1 Evans DH, McDicken WN, Skidmore R, Woodcock JP. (1989) *Doppler Ultrasound: Physics, Instrumentation and Clinical Applications.* Wiley, Chichester.

2 Powis RL, Schwartz RD. (1991) *Practical Doppler Ultrasound for the Clinician.* Williams and Wilkins, Baltimore.

3 Kremkau FW. (1992) Principles and instrumentation. *In: Doppler Color Imaging*, pp. 7–60. Edited by Merritt CRB. Churchill Livingstone, New York.

4 Wells PNT. (1992) Physical and technical aspects of colour flow ultrasound. In: *Diagnostic Vascular Ultrasound*, pp. 145–53. Edited by Labs KH *et al.* Edward Arnold, London.

5 Gill RW. (1985) Measurement of blood flow by ultrasound: accuracy and sources of error. *Ult Med Biol* **11**: 625–42.

6 Rourke C, Hendrickx P, Roth U, Brassel F, Creutzig A, Alexander K. (1992) Color and conventional image-directed ultrasonography: accuracy and sources of error in quantitative blood flow measurement. *J Clin Ultrasound* **20**: 187–93.

7a Thompson RS, Trudinger BJ, Cook CM. (1986) A comparison of Doppler ultrasound waveform indices in the umbilical artery I. Indices derived from the maximum velocity waveform. *Ult Med Biol* **12**: 835–44.

7b Thompson RS, Trudinger BJ, Cook CM. (1986) A comparison of Doppler ultrasound waveform indices in the umbilical artery II. Indices derived from the mean velocity and first moment waveforms. *Ult Med Biol* **12**: 845–54.

8 Planiol T, Pourcelot L. (1973) Doppler effect study of the carotid circulation. In: *Ultrasonics in Medicine*, pp. 104–11. Edited by de Vlieger M, White DN, McCready VR. Elsevier, New York.

9 Gosling RG, King DH. (1974) Continuous wave ultrasound as an alternative and complement to X-rays in vascular examination. In: *Cardiovascular Applications of Ultrasound*, pp. 266–82. Edited by Reneman RS. North-Holland, Amsterdam.

10. Report on WFUMB symposium on safety and standardisation in medical ultrasound. (1992) *Ult Med Biol* **18**(9): 731–809.

11. Duck FA, Starritt HC, ter Haar GR, Lunt MJ. (1989) Surface heating of diagnostic ultrasound transducers. *Br J Rad* **62**: 1005–13.

CHAPTER 2

A practical approach to obtaining optimum Doppler signals

Colin Deane and Kevin Harrington

INTRODUCTION

Before using Doppler ultrasound in a clinical setting, the operator should be familiar with general Doppler principles and the specific features of the machine to be used for imaging. Once confidence is gained in the operation of the machine and in the way it produces images, the user can concentrate on the haemodynamic interpretation of the image and the flow measurements.

Manufacturers have different approaches to control layout, operation and to the nomenclature of functions. Although there may appear to be many controls and

parameters to set up, in practice there are a few steps which make large changes to the quality of the image. Many of the minor controls make only small changes to suit a particular application or the operator's own preference. Manufacturers offer applications/set-up keys which set many of these controls with one keystroke to suit a specific examination.

The following is a general guide to the steps necessary to obtain the optimum signal when conducting a Doppler scan. The first part of the chapter is a guide to factors governing a continuous wave (CW) Doppler-only examination. The second part shows how to set up a colour flow scan, initially using the controls to obtain a colour image and subsequently to produce the PW spectral Doppler sonogram suitable for measurements.

CONTINUOUS WAVE (CW) DOPPLER

1 Choose the probe transmitter frequency appropriate for the examination. High transmitter frequencies give a higher frequency Doppler

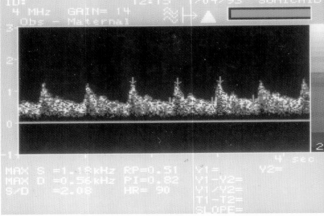

(a)

(b)

Fig. 2.1
(a) The artery is insonated using 8 MHz CW Doppler; peak Doppler frequency is 2.37 kHz. Despite high receiver gain, the Doppler sonogram is of poor quality and there is variation in the computed minimum diastolic velocity over three cycles (calculated PI 1.14). (b) Using 4 MHz CW ultrasound on the same artery, the Doppler shifts are half those for the 8 MHz transducer (peak Doppler frequency now 1.18 kHz). However, the quality of the sonogram is improved and there is more consistency in the computed parameters over three cycles (calculated PI = 0.82).

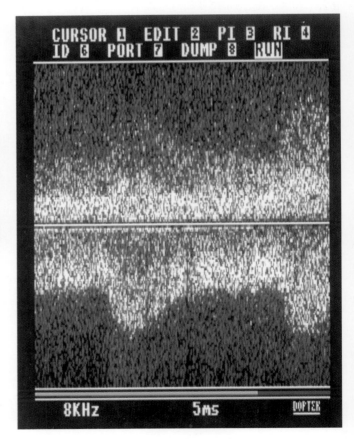

Fig. 2.2
The sonogram has too much receiver gain. The sonogram is ambiguous and there is background noise.

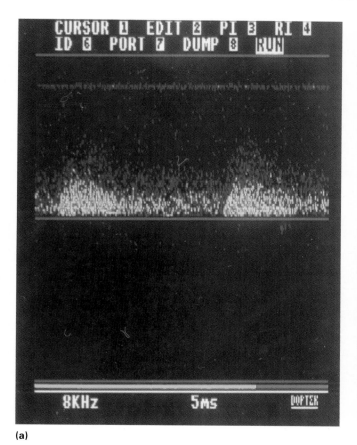
(a)

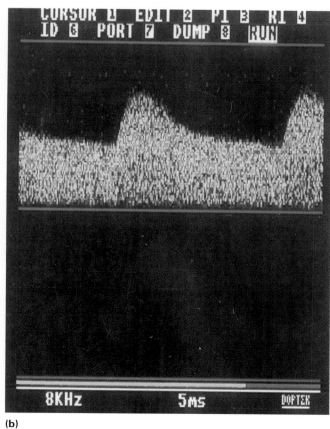
(b)

Fig. 2.3
(a) The sonogram has a low Doppler frequency because of poor beam/flow angle. Accurate calculations are not possible. (b) By moving the probe slightly and insonating the same vessel at an improved beam/flow angle, a clear sonogram suitable for analysis is obtained.

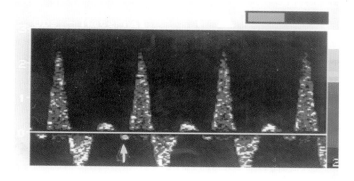
(a)

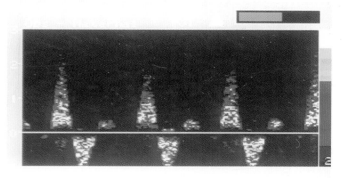
(b)

Fig. 2.5
Using a low frequency wall filter (a), the reverse flow at the end of diastole is observed (arrow). A high frequency wall filter removes this part of the waveform (b).

shift, but the signal quality may be insufficient for analysis because of attenuation (Fig. 2.1).

2 **Adjust the output power and receiver gain to obtain a clear sonogram.** Too much gain results

in extraneous noise in the sonogram (Fig. 2.2). Too little gain produces an inadequate Doppler signal.

3 **Adjust the probe/flow angle to obtain the optimum signal possible.** The Doppler fre-

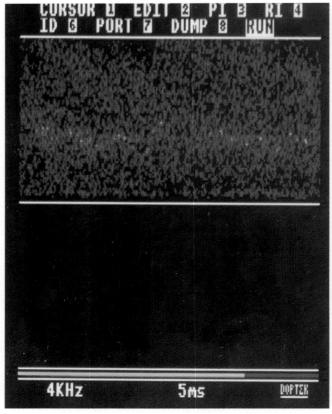

(a)

Fig. 2.4
The y-axis range (4 kHz) is inappropriate for the range of Doppler frequencies in the sonogram. A wider range scale of 8 kHz (Fig. 2.3(b)) should be used.

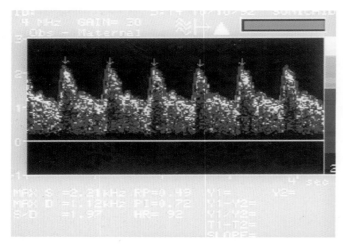

Fig. 2.7
The sonogram signal quality is good. The display axis scales show the sonogram clearly. The heart rate is regular. This is an ideal sonogram from which to make measurements.

quency increases as the beam becomes more aligned with the direction of flow. Try angling the probe or use a different approach if the Doppler frequency shift is low (Fig. 2.3).

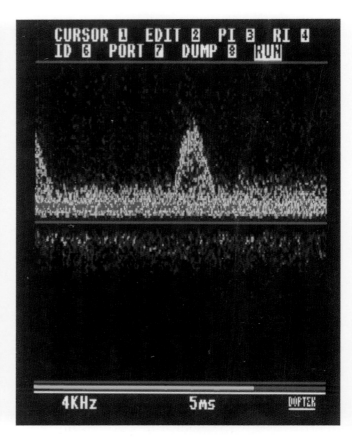

Fig. 2.6
The CW beam insonates an artery and a vein. The venous Doppler signal obscures most of the arterial signal.

4 **Set the time and frequency axes to the appropriate scale** (Fig. 2.4). Adjust the axes so that the screen displays the sonogram to its best advantage.
5 **Set the filter (wall filter) to the appropriate level.** A high frequency filter may reduce noise from tissue movement, but some information in the sonogram is lost (Fig. 2.5).
6 **Avoid insonating multiple vessels.** If measurements and calculations are required from a vessel, the presence of signals from another vessel can lead to errors (Fig. 2.6).
7 **Obtain the sonogram and make the necessary measurements** (Fig. 2.7).

COLOUR DOPPLER IMAGING AND COLOUR VELOCITY IMAGING

Choose the appropriate transducer for the examination. This will be governed by B-mode as well as CDI/CVI and PW spectral Doppler requirements. (Many scanners use transducers which operate at different frequencies for different modes, e.g. 5 MHz for B-mode and 3.5 MHz for CDI and spectral Doppler.)

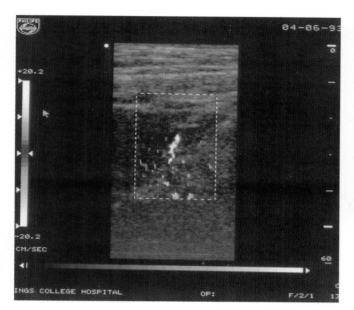

Fig. 2.8
The colour gain is set too high. There are extraneous colour returns from tissue.

Colour flow scan (CDI or CVI)

1 **Select the application/set-up key appropriate for the examination.** This optimizes many of the parameters (e.g. colour map used, colour filter, colour persistence, frame rate/pixel size settings) to suit the chosen investigation. These parameters vary between manufacturers; operators should familiarize themselves with the facilities offered on the machine used. Alterations may be made to these during the examination (some of the changes are described in

Fig. 2.11
Colour aliasing. The colour scale is set low (PRF is low). The aliasing in the colour image of the vessel makes the direction of the flow unclear.

Chapter 1), but many of these parameters can be left unchanged during a specific examination.

2 **Set the transmitted power within safety limits for fetal studies.** Adjust the colour gain to obtain a satisfactory signal from flow regions while excluding signals from surrounding tissue (Fig. 2.8). Ensure that focus/transmit zone is at or near the depth of investigation.

3 **Use probe positioning or beam steering (linear array probes) to obtain a satisfactory beam/vessel angle** (Fig. 2.9).

4 **Set the area under colour flow investigation to the appropriate size.** A reduced colour flow area may increase the frame rate and reduce pixel

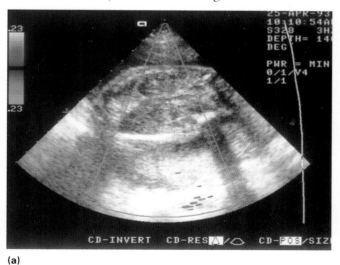

(a)

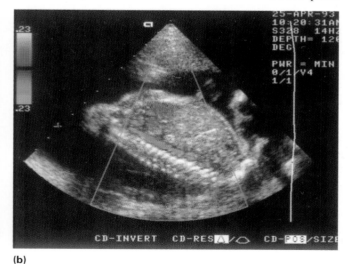

(b)

Fig. 2.9
(a) The fetal aorta lies parallel to the transducer face; the phased array transducer produces both forward (red) and reverse (blue) frequency shifts from flow within it. (b) By changing the approach, the fetal aorta appears clearly with flow away from the transmitted beams. This approach provides a consistent colour image and will provide a better beam/vessel angle for PW spectral Doppler.

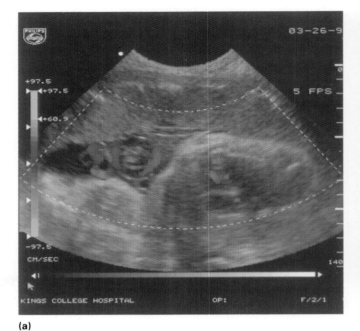

(a)

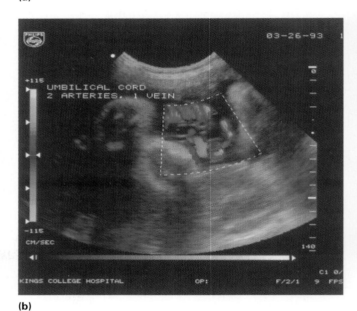

(b)

Fig. 2.10

(a) The area under CVI investigation is large. Frame rate falls to 5 frames per second. (b) By reducing the area under CVI investigation, frame rate improves because fewer colour scan lines are needed (frame rate 9 fps).

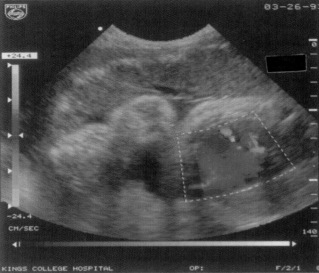

(a)

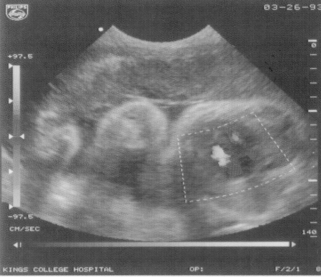

(b)

Fig. 2.12 *Colour scale in CVI.*

(a) With the velocity scale set low, the range of flow velocities arising from the complex flow in the heart obscures detail. (b) With the velocity scale raised, the CVI mode is less sensitive to low flow velocities and the high flow velocities arising from ventricular filling are seen clearly.

size, improving temporal and spatial resolution (Fig. 2.10).

5 **Set the colour scale/PRF and baseline correctly to image the vessels under investigation.** Low PRFs/velocity scales increase sensitivity to low flow velocities but can lead to aliasing of high flow velocities. High PRFs/velo-city scales can reduce aliasing but are less sensitive to low velocities (Figs 2.11 and 2.12).

An example of an optimized colour flow image is shown in Fig. 2.13.

Pulsed wave (spectral) Doppler

1 **Set the transmitted power within safety limits for fetal studies.**
2 **Position the PW Doppler cursor on the vessel to be imaged.** Adjust the Doppler gain to obtain a good quality sonogram with low noise (Fig. 2.14).

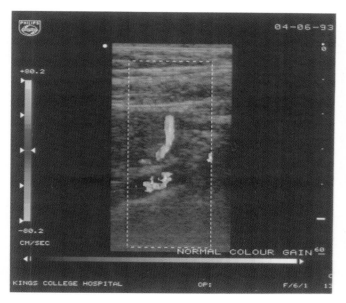

Fig. 2.13
CVI image of a uterine artery. The image is free from extraneous colour signals. The probe and beam are aligned well with the artery to give a good beam/vessel angle. The direction of flow is clear.

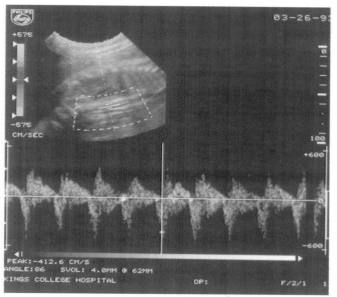

(a)

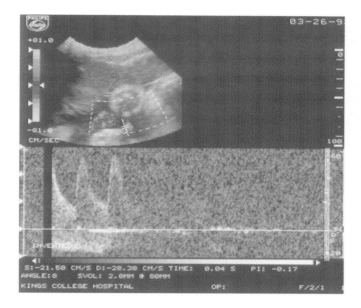

Fig. 2.14
The PW sample volume (gate) is not positioned accurately on the vessel. The Doppler gain is set high to compensate for the poor quality signal. The sonogram is noisy and the arterial signal is soon lost due to breathing movement.

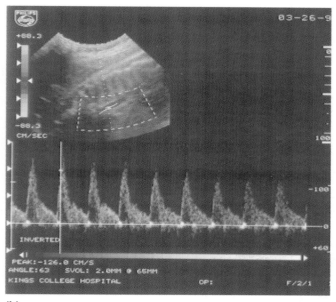

(b)

Fig. 2.15
(a) The high beam/flow angle (86°) results in a confusing sonogram from the vessel under study. (b) By repositioning the probe, a better beam/flow angle (63°) is obtained. The sonogram is unambiguous.

3 **Use beam steering or probe positioning to obtain a satisfactory beam/flow angle.** Angles close to 90° will give ambiguous or unclear sonograms (Fig. 2.15).

4 **Select the appropriate PRF/velocity scale and baseline for the sonogram.** For accurate interpretation and measurement, the PRF and baseline should be chosen so that the sonogram is clearly defined and is not aliased (Figs 2.16 and 2.17).

5 **Make the beam/flow angle correction if velocities are to be derived from the Doppler frequency shift.** Use the B-mode or colour flow image of the vessel to make the angle correction (Fig. 2.18). Without an angle correction, velocities

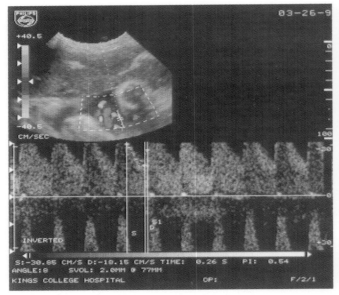

(a)

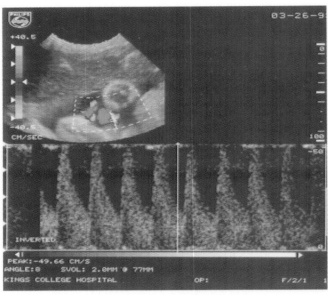

(b)

Fig. 2.16
(a) The velocity scale is set incorrectly for the artery under investigation. High systolic velocities are misinterpreted on the sonogram due to aliasing. (b) By altering the baseline, aliasing no longer occurs and the sonogram is unambiguous.

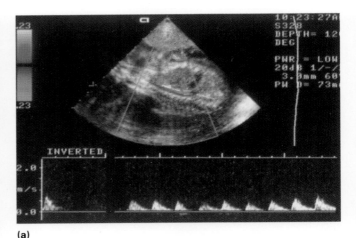

(a)

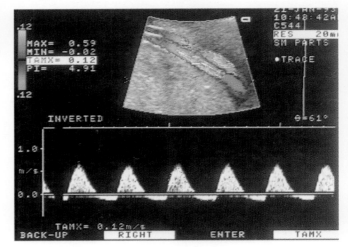

(b)

Fig. 2.17
(a) The velocity scale is not optimized for the low frequency shifts arising from the fetal aorta. Definition of the waveform is poor. (b) By decreasing the velocity scale, the shape of the sonogram is seen more clearly.

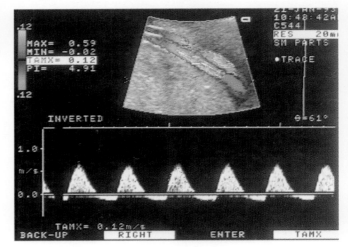

Fig. 2.18
Using the colour image of the vessel, a beam/flow angle correction is made. Velocity scales on the sonogram now accurately reflect arterial velocities.

are incorrect. Even with an angle correction, velocities may still be in error if the beam/flow angle is not measured accurately. The effect of angle error becomes increasingly severe as the beam/flow angle increases.

6 **Set the Doppler sample volume size (gate) to the desired size.** If flow measurements are being attempted, the whole vessel should be insonated (Fig. 2.19). A large gate may include signals from adjacent vessels.

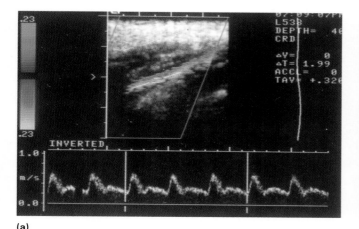

(a)

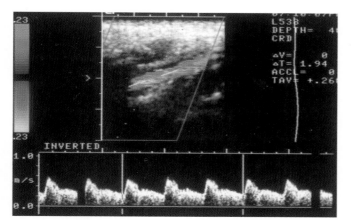

(a)

Fig. 2.19

(a) The sample volume (gate) insonates the centre of the artery only where velocities are highest. The mean velocity across three cardiac cycles is calculated as 32 cm/sec. (b) The sample volume insonates the entire width of the artery including the low velocities near the arterial wall. Calculated mean velocity across three cardiac cycles is 26cm/sec. By using the centre stream velocities (see (a)), the mean velocity in the artery is overestimated.

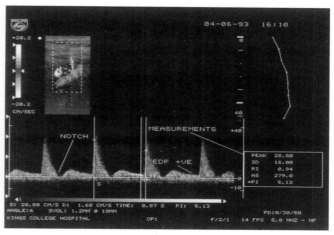

Fig. 2.20

CVI has been used to provide sample volume positioning and beam/vessel angle. The sonogram shows consistency over four cardiac cycles. Measurements of peak velocity, PI, RI, S/D ratio and the presence of a post-systolic notch are made.

7 **If necessary, use the filter to remove low frequency noise due to tissue movement (e.g. wall thump).** Use of a high frequency filter can remove low velocity signals and lead to errors in waveform and velocity measurements.
8 **Make the required measurements from the sonogram** (Fig. 2.20).

SUMMARY

In this chapter, the parameters which affect the Doppler image have been described and their effects shown. With familiarity of equipment used, the Doppler ultrasound user rapidly becomes accustomed to these effects. With practice, controls and scanning approach can be quickly adjusted and the image optimized to provide the best possible information for clinical diagnosis.

CHAPTER 3

Early pregnancy

Bruce Ramsay and Eric Jauniaux

INTRODUCTION

The process of embryonic development has been of great interest to anatomists and biologists for more than a century. In a world in which the study of 'life *in utero*' and antenatal diagnosis of diseases have become realities, research on the pathophysiology of early pregnancy has taken on a new importance and relevance.[1,2] As a result, there is now a reasonable body of scientific evidence supporting a close interaction between the conceptus and mother as early as the blastocyst stage. The placenta and the secondary yolk sac also play fundamental roles in early pregnancy and abnormal development of these organs is associated with subsequent poor outcome.

The two major advances of recent years in the study and management of early pregnancy and its complications have been the widespread introduction of the human chorionic gonadotrophin (β-HCG) assay and transvaginal sonography (TVS). Whilst the ability to diagnose pregnancy biochemically from an early stage is undoubtedly helpful, it offers no anatomical information and can even lead to confusion because β-HCG will remain elevated for some time following pregnancy failure. It is therefore now normal practice to perform an ultrasound examination in all cases of complicated early pregnancy. Previously this examination would have been performed by transabdominal sonography (TAS), but now TVS is the investigation of choice. The probe is closer to the structures under scrutiny and so allows a higher frequency beam to be used which dramatically improves B-mode image resolution. In real terms this means that structures can be visualized a week earlier with TVS than with TAS and also avoids the need for a full bladder.

The subsequent development of vaginal probes with a capability for colour flow imaging has revolutionized our ability to map out the fetal and maternal circulations during the earliest stages of pregnancy.[1,2] From the second month of gestation, colour flow imaging allows identification of the various branches of the uteroplacental circulation[3–5] and most major placental and cord abnormalities can also be diagnosed as early as the end of the first trimester (see Chapter 5).

SITE AND VIABILITY OF EARLY PREGNANCY

During the second and third months of gestation, the developing embryo is enveloped by two fluid compartments: the amniotic cavity and the extraembryonic coelom. The latter contains the secondary yolk sac and is surrounded by the primitive placenta. By the end of

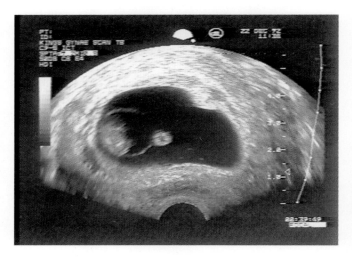

Fig. 3.1
Gestation sac showing amniotic and coelomic cavities

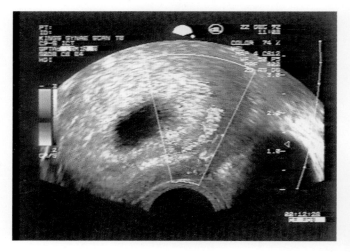

Fig. 3.2
Spiral flow surrounding gestation sac

the first trimester, the enlarging gestational sac fills the entire uterine cavity and fusion of the decidua capsularis and the decidua parietalis obliterates the uterine cavity completely (Fig. 3.1).[2]

The earliest ultrasound sign of pregnancy using conventional scanning is a gestation sac within the uterine cavity. It is eccentric and appears as a double ring.[6] It must be distinguished from the 'pseudogestation sac' that forms in ectopic pregnancy which is a fluid collection due to secretory activity within the uterine cavity seen as a central, single ring structure. Colour Doppler helps make this distinction by showing the increased vascularity surrounding the gestation sac due to the increased flow through the spiral arteries (Fig. 3.2).

If problems arise as pregnancy advances, ultrasound may be used to confirm fetal viability. In this clinical

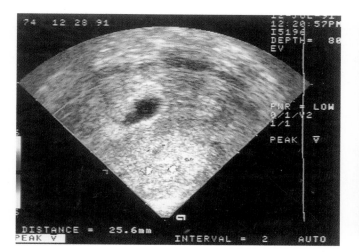

Fig. 3.3
Missed abortion

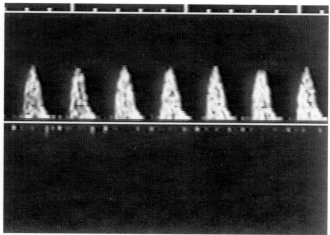

Fig. 3.5
Fetal heart at 10 weeks (rate 170)

Table 3.1 Embryonic/fetal heart rate (mean ± standard deviation) and gestational age of 204 pregnancies from an unselected antenatal population.

Gestation (weeks)	CRL (mm)	n	Mean ± SD (bpm)	Range ± (bpm)
6	0.4–0.9	23	125 ± 15	92–150
7	1.0–1.5	29	146 ± 11	128–161
8	1.6–2.2	24	170 ± 9	151–185
9	2.3–3.0	24	177 ± 7	168–188
10	3.1–4.0	24	172 ± 7	160–186
11	4.1–5.2	23	168 ± 8	158–182
12	5.3–6.6	18	165 ± 6	156–176
13	6.7–7.9	19	164 ± 6	152–170
14	8.0–9.0	20	158 ± 6	150–168

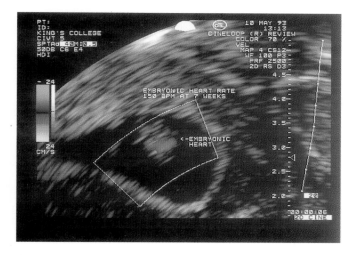

Fig. 3.4
Fetal heart at 6 weeks (rate 125)

situation the embryonic heart pulsation can be seen as early as 35 days from the last menstrual period. Indeed, if there is no heart activity detected by TVS when the embryo crown–rump length is greater than 5 mm, then evidence suggests that the pregnancy is non-viable[7, 8] (Fig. 3.3). Colour Doppler imaging not only makes diagnosis easier in this situation but also provides an excellent visual demonstration for the anxious mother. The ability to make a diagnosis of viability or non-viability on a single scan is not only preferable for the woman concerned but also makes sensible use of limited resources by avoiding repeat visits.

From 6 to 9 weeks of gestation there is a rapid increase of the mean heart rate from 125 to 177 beats per minute (bpm) and this parallels the increase in crown–rump length seen (Figs 3.4 and 3.5). Thereafter the heart rate decreases so by 14 weeks' gestation the

mean is 158 bpm (Table 3.1). The increased heart rate is probably required to increase cardiac output and meet the demands of the growing conceptus at this stage of pregnancy.

Evidence suggests that assessment of the changing embryonic heart rate may be helpful in predicting subsequent pregnancy outcome. A rate of less than 85 bpm on an initial scan between 5 and 7 weeks' gestation[9] or a decreasing rate seen on serial scans[10] are both ominous signs of impending miscarriage. Whilst it is true that chromosomally abnormal fetuses may have an abnormal heart rate,[11] this is an inconsistent finding and not in itself useful as a screening test.[12] However, it has been shown that if the heart rate is abnormal then invasive procedures, such as chorionic villus sampling, should be postponed for 2 weeks.[13] This will avoid unnecessary intervention in cases which are highly likely to miscarry in the near future. If the pregnancy does end in spontaneous miscarriage, an ultrasound diagnosis of an empty uterus can reliably avoid the need for an unnecessary evacuation procedure.[14]

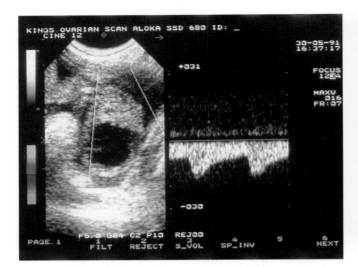

Fig. 3.6
Corpus luteum blood flow

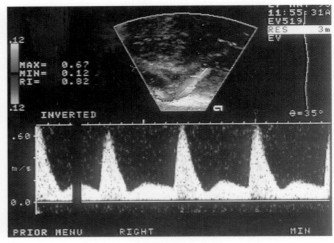

Fig. 3.7
Uterine artery waveform with high RI and notch

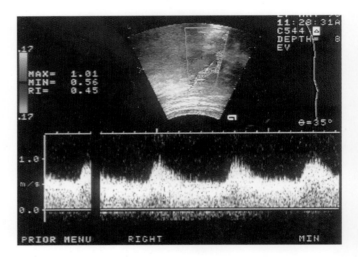

Fig. 3.8
Uterine artery waveform with low RI and no notch

UTERINE AND OVARIAN CIRCULATION

Implantation and the subsequent normal development of an embryo requires considerable adaptive changes to the maternal circulatory system. Anatomical studies have demonstrated that the uterine vascular network elongates and dilates steadily throughout pregnancy.[15] These uterine vascular changes are closely related to the trophoblastic infiltration of the placental bed[16] whilst vessels in the corpus luteum result mainly from a process of independent neoangiogenesis[5] (Fig. 3.6). These specific anatomical differences may explain why there is a significant correlation of gestational age with all Doppler measurements obtained from the uterine circulation but not with those of the corpus luteum.

The fall in uterine vascular resistance is not exclusively due to erosion of the spiral vessels by the invasive trophoblast, since in several animal species it occurs without destruction or invasion of the maternal uterine tissue.[17] In humans, the vascular transformation secondary to placentation is related to variations in circulating oestrogen levels.[18] The similarity of blood flow measurements in both right and left uterine arteries in cases of ectopic pregnancy[19] also supports the view that hormonal factors, such as oestradiol, play a crucial role in regulating the uterine vascular changes. The effect of oestrogen on the general vasculature has already been demonstrated by means of Doppler investigations in post-menopausal women receiving oestrogen replacement therapy.[20, 21]

In the non-pregnant state the uterine artery flow velocity waveform shows low velocities, particularly in diastole, and a post-systolic notch. The calculated indices show a high resistance index (RI) and pulsatility index (PI) with a low mean velocity (Fig. 3.7). With advancing gestation the diastolic velocities increase, the PI and RI fall and the notch disappears (Fig. 3.8). These changes start as early as 8 weeks' gestation and are completed by 20 weeks' gestation in the vast majority of cases.[22] A persistence of the high resistance pattern beyond this time is associated with the subsequent development of pre-eclampsia and intrauterine growth retardation (See Chapter 4).[23]

THE FETAL CIRCULATION

Colour imaging has allowed detailed study of the fetal vasculature from the earliest stages of pregnancy and indeed, most major fetal vessels can be identified by the end of the first trimester. However, whilst trans-

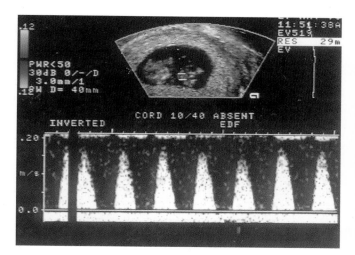

Fig. 3.9
Flow velocity wave form of the umbilical cord at 10 weeks'
gestation, with absent EDF

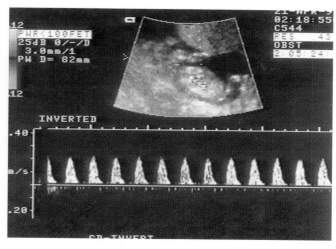

Fig. 3.11
Flow velocity wave form of the fetal aorta at 10 weeks'
gestation, with absent EDF

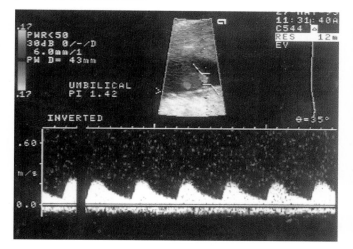

Fig. 3.10
Flow velocity wave form of the umbilical cord at 18 weeks'
gestation, with positive EDF

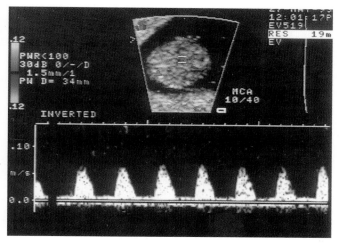

Fig. 3.12
Flow velocity wave form of the fetal intracerebral vessel at 10
weeks' gestation, with absent EDF

vaginal colour Doppler allows signals to be obtained
from these vessels, the clinical value of such investigations remains to be defined.

The umbilical cord pulsations are easily measured
and show absent end diastolic flow (EDF) up to the
end of the first trimester[24] (Fig. 3.9). After this time
diastolic velocities increase progressively and are
universally present after 18 weeks (Fig. 3.10). The fetal
aorta shows a very similar pattern of development to
that of the umbilical cord with the appearance of diastolic velocities occurring during the second trimester
(Fig. 3.11). The PI falls during the first 16 weeks but
then remains relatively constant throughout the rest of
pregnancy.[24]

Intracranial blood flow first becomes visible using
transvaginal colour Doppler from 8 weeks' gestation (Fig. 3.12). End diastolic velocities develop more
rapidly in the intracranial circulation than in other parts
of the fetus and positive EDF is universally present by
14 weeks' gestation (Fig. 3.13).[25] The calculated indices
derived from the waveform also change rapidly during
the early stages of pregnancy so that the PI falls with
increasing gestation. The carotid artery may be visualized separately late in the first trimester but waveforms
obtained vary little from those of other intracerebral
vessels (Fig. 3.14). Doppler studies of intracerebral flow
at the end of the first trimester do not appear helpful in
predicting subsequent poor pregnancy outcome.[25]

Characteristic intracardiac waveforms can be identified from early in the second trimester. The E (early
diastolic filling) and A (atrial contraction) waves can be
measured across both mitral and tricuspid valves. The

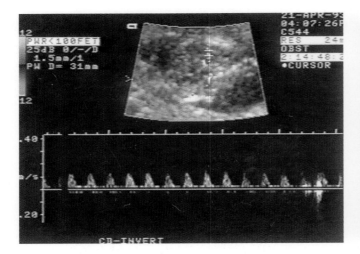

Fig. 3.13
Flow velocity wave form of a fetal intracerebral vessel at 12 weeks' gestation, with positive EDF

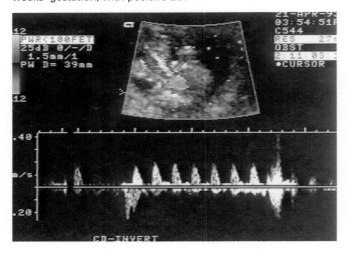

Fig. 3.14
Flow velocity wave form of a fetal cartoid artery

E/A ratio relates the passive to the active phase of ventricular filling. This ratio increases during pregnancy from 0.5 in the first trimester to 0.9 at term and this probably reflects the increasing ventricular compliance which develops with advancing gestation.[24]

The poor ventricular compliance in early pregnancy is also shown by the sharp deceleration of velocities during atrial contraction ('a' wave) (Fig. 3.15). Compare this with ductus venosus flow later in pregnancy (Chapter 7, the venous circulation).

SUMMARY

The first trimester of pregnancy is a fascinating stage of human development *in utero*. Anatomically, it is the time of organogenesis, degeneration of the secondary yolk sac, closure of the exocoelomic cavity, fusion of

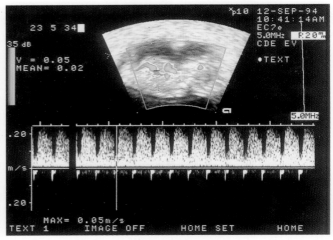

Fig. 3.15
Flow velocity waveform obtained from the ductus venosus in the first trimester. The large deceleration in velocities seen during atrial contraction ('a' wave) reflects the poor compliance of the fetal heart in early pregnancy. Figure courtesy of Dr N. Zosmer

the decidua capsularis and decidua parietalis, disappearance of two-thirds of the placental mass and structural modification of the uteroplacental circulation. Physiologically, there is no true maternal circulation inside the placenta before 12 weeks and the villous barrier is 4–5 times thicker than in the third trimester. Colour Doppler ultrasound has allowed detailed study of the developing circulation and has yielded much valuable information concerning the physiology of early human pregnancy.

REFERENCES

1 Jauniaux E, Jurkovic D, Campbell S, Kurjak A, Hustin J. (1991) Investigation of placental circulations by colour Doppler ultrasound. *Am J Obstet Gynecol* **164**: 486–8.

2 Jauniaux E, Jurkovic D, Campbell S. (1991) In vivo investigations of the anatomy and the physiology of early human placental circulations. *Ultrasound Obstet Gynecol* **1**: 435–45.

3 Jurkovic D, Jauniaux E, Kurjak A, Hustin J, Campbell S, Nicolaides KH. (1991) Transvaginal colour Doppler assessment of utero-placental circulation in early pregnancy. *Obstet Gynaecol* **77**: 365–9.

4 Jaffe R, Warsof SL. (1991) Transvaginal colour Doppler imaging in the assessment of uteroplacental blood flow in the normal first-trimester pregnancy. *Am J Obstet Gynecol* **164**: 781–5.

5 Jurkovic D, Jauniaux E, Campbell S. (1992) Doppler ultrasound investigation of pelvic circulation during the menstrual cycle and early pregnancy. In: *The*

First Twelve Weeks of Gestation, pp. 78–96. Edited by Barnea E, Hustin J, Jauniaux E. Springer-Verlag, Heidelberg.

6 Neiman HL. (1990) Transvaginal ultrasound embryography. *Sem Ultrasound, CT, NMR* **11**: 22–33.

7 Levi CS, Lyons EA, Zheng XH, Lindsay DJ, Holt SC. (1990) Endovaginal ultrasound: Demonstration of cardiac activity in embryos of less than 5.0 mm in crown–rump length. *Radiology* **176**: 71–4.

8 Brown DL, Emerson DS, Felker RE, Cartier MS, Chapman Smith W. (1990) Diagnosis of early embryonic demise by endovaginal sonography. *J Ult Med* **9**: 631–6.

9 May DA, Sturtevant NV. (1991) Embryonic heart rate as a predictor of pregnancy outcome: A prospective analysis. *J Ult Med* **10**: 591–3.

10 Merchiers EH, Dhont M, De Sutter PA, Beghin CJ, Vandekerckhove DA. (1991) Predictive value of early embryonic cardiac activity for pregnancy outcome. *Am J Obstet Gynecol* **165**: 11–14.

11 Schats R, Jansen CAM, Wladimiroff JW. (1990) Abnormal embryonic heart rate pattern in early pregnancy associated with Down's syndrome. *Hum Reprod* **7**: 877–9.

12 Van Lith JMM, Visser GHA, Mantingh A, Beekhuis JR. (1992) Fetal heart rate in early pregnancy and chromosonal disorders. *Br J Obstet Gynaecol* **99**: 741–4.

13 Yagel S, Anteby E, Ron M, Hochner-Celnikier D. (1992) The role of abnormal fetal heart rate in scheduling chorionic villus sampling. *Br J Obstet Gynaecol* **99**: 739–40.

14 Rulin MC, Bornstein SG, Campbell JD. (1993) The reliability of ultrasonography in the management of spontaneous abortion, clinically thought to be complete: A prospective study. *Am J Obstet Gynecol* **168**: 12–15.

15 Ramsey EM, Donner NW. (1980) *Placental Vasculature and Circulation*. Georg Thieme, Stuttgart.

16 Brossens I, Robertson WB, Dixon HG. (1967) The physiological response of the vessels of the placental bed to normal pregnancy. *J Path Bact* **93**: 569–79.

17 Burton GJ. (1992) Human and animal models: Limitations and comparisons. In: *The First Twelve Weeks of Gestation*, pp. 469–85. Edited by Barnea E, Hustin J, Jauniaux E. Springer-Verlag, Heidelberg.

18 Jauniaux E, Jurkovic D, Delogne-Desnoek J, Meuris S. (1992) Influence of human chorionic gonadotrophin, oestradiol and progesterone on uteroplacental and corpus luteum blood flow in normal early pregnancy. *Hum Repro* **7**: 1467–73.

19 Jurkovic D, Bourne TH, Jauniaux E, Campbell S, Collins WP. (1992) Doppler study of blood flow in ectopic pregnancies. *Fertil Steril* **57**: 68–73.

20 De Ziegler D, Bessis R, Frydman R. (1991) Vascular resistance of uterine arteries: physiological effects of estradiol and progesterone. *Fertil Steril* **55**: 775–9.

21 Gangar KF, Vyas S, Whitehead M, Crook D, Meire H, Campbell S. (1991) Pulsatility index in internal carotid artery in relation to transdermal oestradiol and time of menopause. *Lancet* **338**: 839–42.

22 Jauniaux E, Jurkovic D, Campbell S, Hustin J. (1992) Doppler ultrasonographic features of the developing placental circulations: Correlation with anatomic findings. *Am J Obstet Gynecol* **166**: 585–7.

23 Bewley S, Cooper D, Campbell S. (1991) Doppler investigation of uteroplacental blood flow resistance in the second trimester: a screening study for pre-eclampsia and intrauterine growth retardation. *Br J Obstet Gynaecol* **98**: 871–9.

24 Huisman TWA, Stewart PA, Wladimiroff JW. (1992) Doppler assessment of the normal early fetal circulation. *Ultrasound Obstet Gynecol* **2**: 300–5.

25 Kurjak A, Predanic M, Kupesic-Urek S, Funduk-Kurjak B, Demarin V, Salihagic A. (1992) Transvaginal color Doppler study of middle cerebral artery blood flow in early normal and abnormal pregnancy. *Ultrasound Obstet Gynecol* **2**: 424–8.

CHAPTER 4

The uterine circulation in pregnancy

Kevin Harrington and Stuart Campbell

INTRODUCTION

In the first half of pregnancy the placental trophoblast invades into the myometrium and establishes a low resistance circulation.[1, 2] Proteinuric pregnancy induced hypertension (PPIH)/pre-eclampsia is a common cause of intrauterine growth retardation (IUGR),[3] and is associated with significant maternal and perinatal morbidity and mortality.[4] Primiparous and black women[5] are at greater risk of developing the condition. The aetiology of pre-eclampsia and associated IUGR is thought to lie in a failure of the placenta to establish an adequate circulation within the uterus to supply the growing fetoplacental unit. Partial failure of this process has been linked with subsequent impairment and deterioration of placental function,[6, 7] when fetoplacental demand exceeds placental capacity. Consequently patients usually present with PPIH and/or IUGR in the second half of pregnancy but the pathophysiological changes that lead to this condition develop much earlier.

Doppler ultrasound allows non-invasive investigation of the uteroplacental circulation.[8] Abnormal flow velocity waveforms (FVW) in the uterine arteries recorded by this technique are associated with PPIH[9] and IUGR.[10]

It is the introduction of colour flow/pulsed Doppler duplex systems and endovaginal transducers that has allowed us to build a picture of the physiological changes in uterine blood flow before and during pregnancy. This in turn has led to a greater understanding of the pathological changes seen in the uterine circulation and has refocused attention on Doppler studies of the uterine artery as a potentially useful tool for the prediction of subsequent complications in pregnancy associated with inadequate placentation.

The finding that low dose aspirin, if given early in pregnancy, may ameliorate or abolish the complications associated with incomplete trophoblastic invasion has made the search for a reliable method of predicting such at-risk patients all the more important.[11, 12] The first part of this chapter will illustrate how uterine artery flow velocity waveforms are obtained and describe the physiological changes seen in the uterine circulation during pregnancy. The second part will illustrate how Doppler studies of the uterine artery can be utilized as a test capable of selecting a group at risk of subsequently developing pre-eclampsia and/or an SGA fetus.

OBTAINING DOPPLER MEASUREMENTS FROM THE UTERINE CIRCULATION

The transvaginal and transabdominal approach

The uterine artery is a branch of the internal iliac artery. It courses along the lateral wall of the pelvis before crossing the external iliac artery and reaching the uterus at the level of the cervix (Fig. 4.1). After giving off a cervical branch it ascends along the lateral wall of the body of the uterus in a tortuous manner, before anastomosing with the Fallopian branch of the ovarian artery (Fig. 4.2). As it passes along the body of the uterus it gives off the arcuate arteries which encompass the uterine body and in turn give off radial arteries that penetrate into the inner third of the myometrium, where they become the basal arteries. The spiral arteries, a continuation of the basal arteries, supply the endometrium, their coiled form allowing contraction during menstruation.

Using a transvaginal probe, it is possible to identify

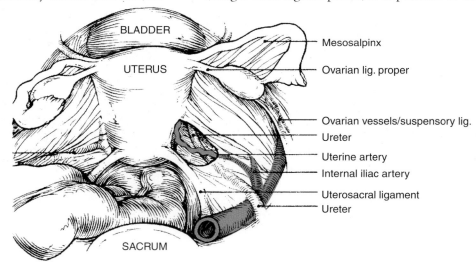

Fig. 4.1
An anatomical diagram of the uterine artery. After branching from the internal iliac artery it courses along the lateral wall of the pelvis before crossing the external iliac artery and reaching the uterus at the level of the cervix.

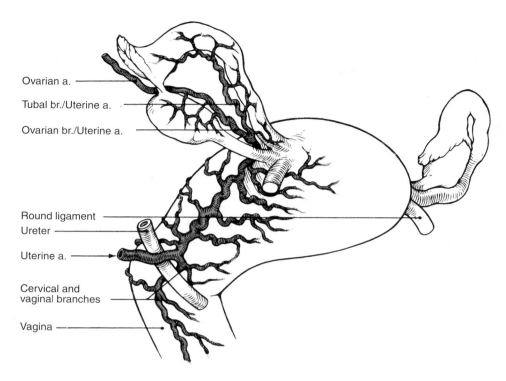

Ovarian a.

Tubal br./Uterine a.

Ovarian br./Uterine a.

Round ligament

Ureter

Uterine a.

Cervical and vaginal branches

Vagina

Fig. 4.2
After giving off a cervical branch the uterine artery ascends along the lateral wall of the body of the uterus in a tortuous manner, before anastomosing with the fallopian branch of the ovarian artery. As it passes along the body of the uterus it gives off the arcuate arteries which encompass the uterine body and in turn give off radial arteries that penetrate into the inner third of the myometrium, where they become the basal arteries.

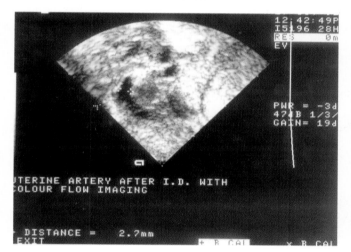

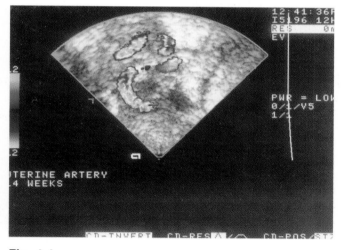

Fig. 4.3
A transvaginal scan showing the vascular plexus that surrounds the cervix. After identifying the cervix, if the transducer is moved laterally, the vascular plexus will become visible

Fig. 4.4
When colour flow mapping is applied to the same image (Fig.4.3) the uterine artery is clearly distinguished from the venous vessels by the bright colours and winding path along the lateral wall of the uterus

the uterine artery at the level of the cervical os, as it enters the uterus, and as it ascends into the uterine body (Fig. 4.3). With CDI it is possible to differentiate the uterine artery from the venous plexus in this area and also to see its sinuous path, often likened to a

glowing worm (Fig. 4.4). It is possible to obtain a good angle of insonation at this point and the flow velocity waveforms obtained from the uterine artery do not significantly change from entering the uterus up to the point that it reaches the body of the uterus. It is im-

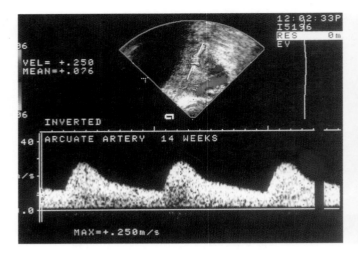

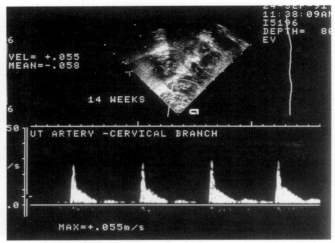

(a)

Fig. 4.5

It is important to examine the uterine artery before the vessel enters the body of the uterus, as it is then indistinguishable from an arcuate artery, shown here. An arcuate artery can exhibit a relatively low resistance waveform even when the main uterine artery is high resistance with persistent notching present. It is necessary, therefore, to ensure that the uterine artery is being examined at the level of the cervix to interpret changes in the uterine circulation as a whole.

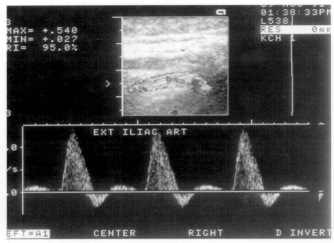

(a)

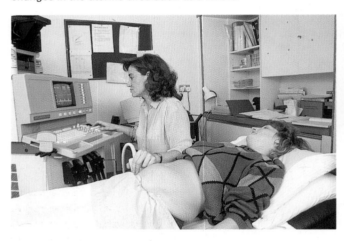

Fig. 4.7

(Photograph of transducer on abdomen for uterine artery measurement.) The transducer should be placed longitudinally in the iliac fossa (right or left, depending on which vessel is being examined). With continuous wave Doppler the probe should be moved in a medial, then lateral direction until the waveform of the uterine artery is obtained.

Fig. 4.6

If the range gate is placed too low on the cervix it is possible to obtain the cervical branch of the uterine artery (a), which can be high resistance when the main uterine artery wave form is normal. The external iliac artery (b) has a characteristic waveform, and with colour flow imaging it should be easily distinguished from the uterine artery.

portant to obtain the measurement at this level, before the uterine artery enters the body of the uterus and has branched into arcuate arteries (Fig. 4.5). If the sample site is too low on the cervix, the cervical branch will be examined by mistake (Fig. 4.6a). With colour flow imaging it should be possible to distinguish the external iliac artery waveform (Fig. 4.6b) even from the uterine waveform.

It is possible to examine the uterine artery by the

transabdominal approach after 12 weeks' gestation, when the uterus becomes an abdominal organ. By placing the transducer in the relevant iliac fossa (Fig. 4.7), it is possible with CDI to follow the course of the uterine artery from the lateral pelvic wall across the external iliac artery onto the cervix and up the lateral wall of the uterus (Fig. 4.8). Pulsed Doppler can then be accurately applied to obtain a FVW (Fig. 4.9). With CW Doppler it is possible to obtain the same waveform, although there is always the possibility of insonating the arcuate artery, which may be of similar appearance but gives a misleading result (Fig. 4.10). This must be kept in mind when using CW Doppler ultra-

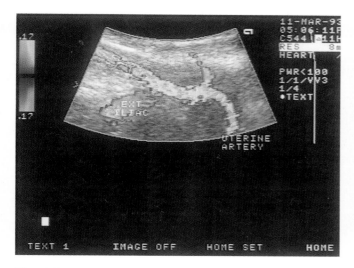

Fig. 4.8
With the transducer placed in the relevant iliac fossa (Fig 4.7), it is now possible to obtain a CDI image of the uterine artery as it crosses the external iliac artery and joins the uterus at the level of the cervix

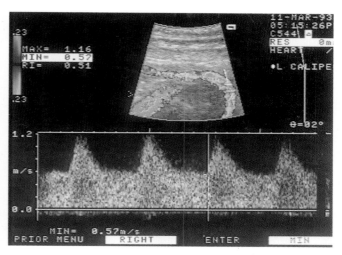

Fig. 4.9
Having located the artery, a pulsed Doppler range gate can be positioned correctly, and a flow velocity waveform obtained. This image shows a normal waveform from a pregnant patient, with abundant diastolic flow.

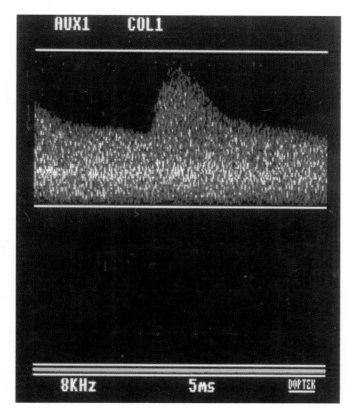

Fig. 4.10
Usually it is easy to find the uterine artery with CW Doppler when blood flow is normal. It can be more difficult when there is abnormal or reduced flow. In this situation the arcuate artery may be insonated by mistake. If there is any doubt as to the vessel being insonated, it is advisable to use CDI to obtain the correct FVW.

sound. If the uterine artery is not found or there is any doubt with CW Doppler ultrasound, it is important to check with CDI/pulsed Doppler as the uterine arteries with the least amount of flow are the most difficult to find with CW Doppler ultrasound.

The uteroplacental circulation – physiological changes during pregnancy

Although actual measurement of volume flow changes in an organ would be ideal, *in vivo* the current methods for determining volume flow are too inaccurate. Consequently we rely on indices of resistance derived from the flow velocity waveform (FVW) and velocity changes of a vessel to give us information on changes in the haemodynamics of a particular organ, in this instance the uterus. Transvaginal ultrasound probes that allow Doppler imaging have enabled us to accurately identify changes in the uterine circulation during the menstrual cycle (Fig. 4.11),[13] and in early pregnancy.[14] With colour Doppler imaging to ensure that the uterine artery is being examined when performing a transabdominal scan, it is possible to map changes in blood flow and resistance from the non-pregnant state and for the duration of the pregnancy. The typical uterine waveform in a non-pregnant patient is shown in Fig. 4.11. The characteristic shape of this waveform shows a steep systolic slope, an early diastolic notch and a small amount of diastolic flow. Although the waveform changes in the menstrual cycle, with more flow in the luteal phase of the cycle, the waveform remains essentially high resistance in the non-pregnant state.

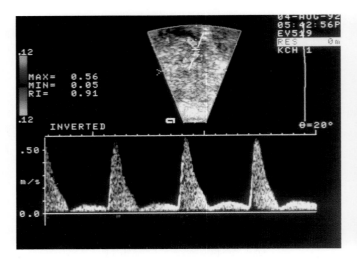

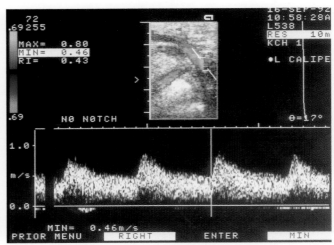

Fig. 4.11

A flow velocity waveform (FVW) obtained from a uterine artery in a non-pregnant patient. The characteristic shape of this waveform shows a steep systolic slope, an early diastolic notch, and a small amount of diastolic flow. Although the waveform changes in the menstrual cycle, with more flow in the luteal phase, the waveform remains essentially high resistance in the non-pregnant state.

Fig. 4.12

FVW in established pregnancy at 20 weeks. Placentation typically results in a low resistance FVW, the disappearance of the notch and an abundance of diastolic flow (compare with the FVW from the non-pregnant patient in Fig 4.11) Failure of this physiological modification is associated with the development of pre-eclampsia and intrauterine growth retardation.

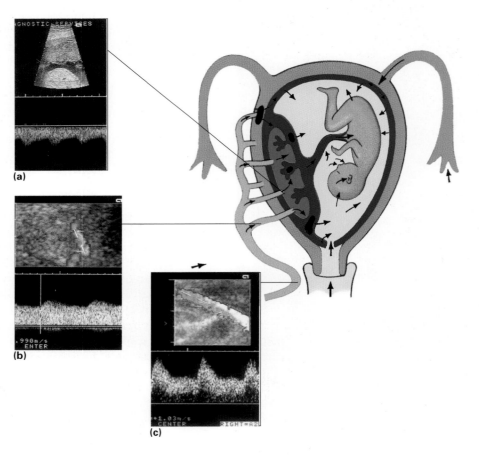

Fig. 4.13

An illustration of uterine blood flow in an established normal pregnancy. The flow waveform in the uterine artery (c) has lost the notch, and end diastolic flow is increased (decreased RI). The arcuate arteries (b) show a more obvious increase in diastolic flow, as do the sub-placental or peritrophoblastic arteries (a).

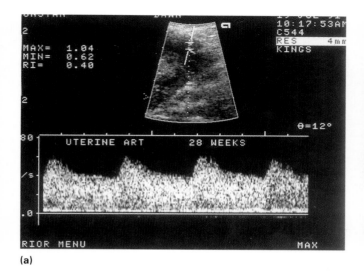

(a)

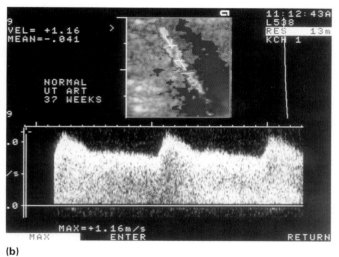

(b)

Fig. 4.14
A normal FVW from the uterine artery at 24 (a) and 38 (b) weeks. About 9% of the population will have persistent notching by 24 weeks. There are further minor changes in the uterine waveform in the last trimester of pregnancy, with some waveforms losing the notch, and others continuing to increase diastolic flow. The predictive value of persistent notching appears to lie earlier in pregnancy, between 16 and 24 weeks.

From very early on in pregnancy, the effect of pregnancy, and in particular placentation, can be seen in the uterine artery waveforms of some patients. As the pregnancy progresses, there is gradual removal of the notch and an increase in diastolic flow, as seen by the fall in the resistance index (RI) (Fig. 4.12). There is also a dramatic rise in the mean velocity of blood flow in the uterine vessels, especially towards the end of the first trimester, at 12–15 weeks. Changes in the rest of the uterine circulation in early pregnancy are illustrated in Fig. 4.13.

By the 20th week of pregnancy the majority of patients have low resistance uterine artery FVWs with

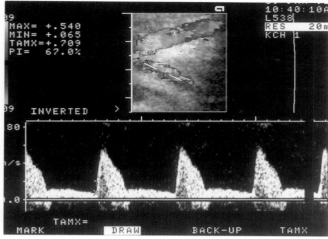

Fig. 4.15
A FVW from the uterine artery in a post partum patient, showing the typical non-pregnant waveform reappearing.

20% retaining a notch in either uterine artery FVW. At 24 weeks the number of patients with notching is 9%. There is little change in the uterine Doppler indices in the third trimester (Fig. 4.14).[15] The uterine artery FVW returns to normal in the first few days after birth (Fig. 4.15). The normal range for the RI of the uterine artery in pregnancy is presented in the Appendix.

DOPPLER ULTRASOUND OF THE UTERINE ARTERY IN THE PREDICTION OF PRE-ECLAMPSIA AND INTRAUTERINE GROWTH RETARDATION

When applying CW Doppler ultrasound to unselected populations the results confirm the value of uterine Doppler studies in identifying high risk pregnancies, but the sensitivity and predictive value of the investigation vary.[16–18] This variation can be explained in part because of differences in the timing, site and evaluation of Doppler studies, by the different equipment used, by the assorted definitions regarding an abnormal outcome to the pregnancy and because it is not always possible to ensure that the uterine artery is being examined when using CW Doppler ultrasound. The complex nature of the uterine circulation and the effect of the placental site has also created differences in the interpretation of Doppler waveforms (Fig. 4.16).[19, 20]

When using the RI alone or as part of an averaged resistance index (AVRI) to screen low risk populations the sensitivity was poor (15% for IUGR, 23% for pre-eclampsia) but the risk of developing any severe complication was 9.8 times higher in patients with an

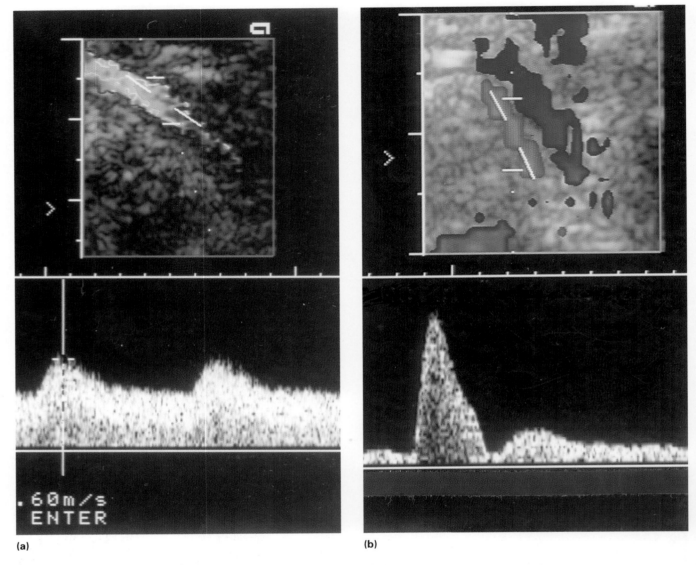

(a)   (b)

Fig. 4.16
FVWs from the right (a) and left (b) uterine artery in a patient with a lateral placenta. The high resistance on one side is balanced by the very low resistance on the other side, suggesting that it is the site rather than the process of implantation that is responsible for the persistent notching.

RI > 95th centile (Fig. 4.17).[21] The predictive value was greater with increasing gestation, but the sensitivity remained low (36%). The strong relationship between an elevated index of resistance and a poor outcome of pregnancy was established, but the poor sensitivity minimizes the potential impact of the AVRI or RI as a screening tool.

Persistent notching of the uterine waveform at 20 and 24 weeks

In view of the limitations of the uterine RI, it was decided to investigate the use of persistent notching of the uterine arteries as the definition of abnormality (Fig. 4.18). This is a simplification of the frequency index profile,[9] which had been found to persist in the majority of patients diagnosed with pre-eclampsia.[17]

CW Doppler studies were performed by the staff on over 2500 women as part of the routine booking ultrasound scans at 19–21 weeks' gestation. If there was persistent notching at this time (Fig. 4.19), the patient was referred for a repeat scan at 24 weeks. Colour Doppler imaging (CDI) was then used to identify the uterine artery, where it crosses over the external iliac artery (Fig. 4.20). This 'cross-over' can be used as a reference point to repeatedly identify the main uterine artery at the same site, thus removing any doubts that exist with

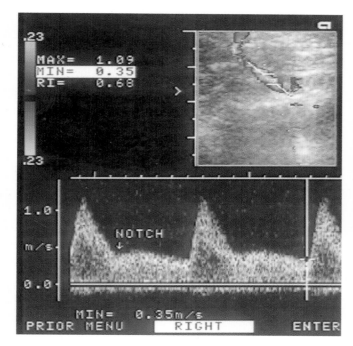

Fig. 4.17
The RI measured in this figure = 0.68. Although there is a strong relationship between an abnormal RI and a poor outcome to pregnancy, the low sensitivity of this test limits its use as a screening test.

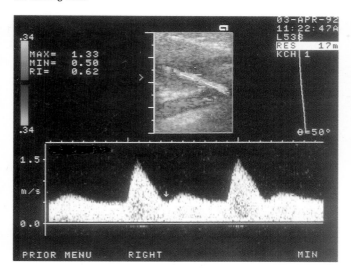

Fig. 4.18
Using CW Doppler a uterine artery FVW obtained at 20 weeks' gestation, showing persistent notching. About 15% of the population will have persistent notching of the uterine artery FVW at 20 weeks whereas approximately 20% of the population will have persistent notching if CDI is employed. Although the specificity is not as high as at 24 weeks, the sensitivity is equally impressive. This group of women contain most of the patients that will subsequently develop pre-eclampsia, and about half the patients that will deliver a small-for-gestational-age baby. It is important to note that uterine artery Doppler is a screening test, not a diagnostic test. Some pregnancies with persistent notching will have a normal outcome to their pregnancy.

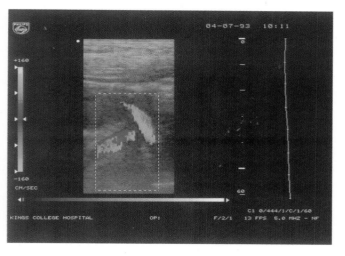

Fig. 4.19
CDI image of the uterine artery as it crosses the external iliac artery. This is a suitable point to place the range gate to obtain the FVW; it is a point that can be identified in most patients, and allows measurement of the uterine artery before it branches into arcuate arteries.

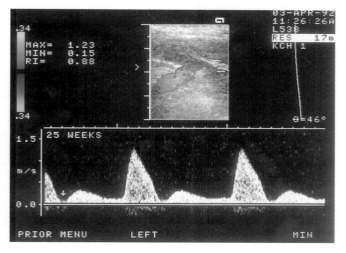

Fig. 4.20
Notch at 25 weeks. An abnormal FVW of the uterine artery at 25 weeks. Persistent notching at 25 weeks implies incomplete trophoblastic invasion, and is predictive of pre-eclampsia. Patients with notching in both uterine arteries at 24 weeks have a one in two chance of developing pre-eclampsia and/or delivering a small-for-gestational-age fetus.

the use of the CW Doppler.[22]

In the study by Bower *et al.*[23] 15% of the population had abnormal waveforms at 19–21 weeks and these were retained by 5% of the patients at 24–26 weeks' gestation (Fig. 4.20). Using persistent notching as the definition of abnormality, the sensitivity compared to the RI dramatically improved (76 *vs* 23%) for the prediction of PPIH, but with a reduced specificity at 20 weeks (95 *vs* 86%). However, the specificity had

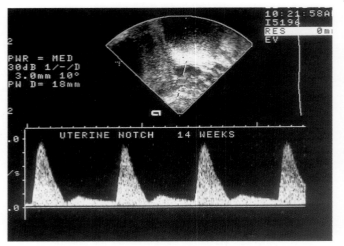

(a)

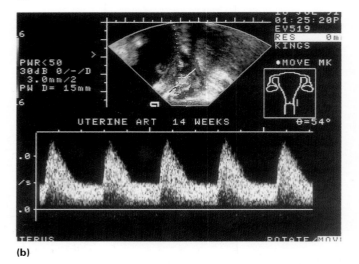

(b)

Fig. 4.21
Uterine artery FVWs obtained with an endovaginal transducer, with (a) and (b) without notching. Over 95% of the patients that will subsequently develop pre-eclamp[sia have persistent notching in both uterine arteries at this stage in the pregnancy.

achieved the same value as the first study[21] by 24–26 weeks (96%).[23]

Persistent notching of the uterine waveform at 13–15 weeks

More recent studies have evaluated the ability of transvaginal Doppler ultrasound of uterine circulation in early pregnancy to predict those patients that would develop pre-eclampsia, IUGR, placental abruption.[24] The uterine arteries were identified with colour flow imaging at the level of the cervical internal os. Pulsed Doppler was then applied to each artery and measurements obtained from a consistent, clear waveform.

From 6 to 16 weeks there is a gradual rise in vessel diameter, mean and maximum velocity, with a concomitant reduction in the resistance index and pulsatility index. There is a fall in the number of bilateral uterine notches from 74% to 38% (Fig. 4.21b). All but one of the patients that subsequently developed pre-eclampsia had persistent notching of at least one uterine artery and nearly all had bilateral notching, with a mean RI>50th centile (Fig. 4.21a).

This adds weight to the hypothesis that the process of placentation is flawed from the beginning of implantation and it is probable that patients with high resistance uterine artery FVWs in the non-pregnant state are at greater risk of developing PPIH compared to women with low resistance waveforms. This suggests ineffective placentation is a problem of both the seed and soil. The excellent sensitivity of persistent bilateral notching (>90%) is tempered by the poor specificity (70%) at this gestation.

SUMMARY

The addition of CDI and transvaginal ultrasound allows us to examine the uterine artery at various gestations. The definition of abnormality being based upon the finding of persistent notching yields a high sensitivity, with a specificity that varies according to the gestation at the time of examination. This holds out the possibility of clinicians being able to utilize this information in clinical practice, especially as a tool for identifying patients that would be suitable for prophylactic treatment with therapies such as low dose aspirin.[25, 26]

REFERENCES

1 Maini CL, Galli G, Bellati U, Bonettie G, Moneta E. (1985) Non-invasive radioisotopic evaluation of placental blood flow. *Gynaecol Obstet Invest* **19**: 196–204

2 Pijnenborg R, Dixon G, Robertson WB, Brosens I. (1980) Trophoblastic invasion of human decidua from 8–18 weeks of pregnancy. *Placenta* **1**: 3–19.

3 Davey DA, MacGillivray I. (1988) The classification and definition of hypertensive disorders of pregnancy. *Am J Obstet Gynecol* **158**: 892–985.

4 Turnbull AC. (1987) Maternal mortality and present trends. In: *Hypertension in Pregnancy*, Proceedings of the Sixteenth Study Group of the Royal College of Obstetricians and Gynaecologists, pp. 155-80. Edited by Sharp F, Symonds EM. Perinatology Press, Oxford.

5 Eskenazi B, Fenster L, Sidney S. (1991) A multivariate analysis of risk factors for pre-eclampsia. *JAMA* **266**: 237–41.

6 Brosens I, Robertson WB, Dixon HG. (1967) The physiological response of the vessels of the placental bed to normal pregnancy. *J Pathol Bacteriol* **93**: 569–79.

7 Khong TY, De Wolf F, Robertson WB, Brosens I. (1986) Inadequate maternal vascular response to placentation in pregnancies complicated by pre-eclampsia and by small-for-gestational age infants. *Br J Obstet Gynaecol* **93**: 1049–59.

8 Stuart B, Drumm J, Fitzgerald D, Duignan NM. (1980) Fetal blood velocity waveforms in normal pregnancy. *Br J Obstet Gynaecol* **88**: 865–9.

9 Campbell S, Diaz-Recasens J, Griffen DR *et al.* (1983) New Doppler technique for assessing uteroplacental blood flow. *Lancet* **1**: 675–77.

10 McCowan LM, Ritchie K, Mo LY, Bascom PA, Sherret H. (1988) Uterine artery flow velocity waveforms in normal and growth retarded pregnancies. *Am J Obstet Gynecol* **158**: 499–504.

11 Beaufils M, Uzan S, Donsimoni R, Colau JC. (1985) Prevention of pre-eclampsia by early antiplatelet therapy. *Lancet* **1**: 840–2.

12 Uzan S, Beaufils M, Breart G, Bazin B, Capitant C, Paris J. (1991) Prevention of fetal growth retardation with low dose aspirin: Findings of the EPREDA trial. *Lancet* **337**: 1427–31.

13 Steer CV, Campbell S, Pampiglione J, Kingsland C, Mason BA, Collins WP. (1990) Transvaginal colour flow imaging of the uterine arteries during the ovarian and menstrual cycles. *Hum Reprod* **5**: 391–9.

14 Jurkovic D, Jauniaux E, Kurjak A, Campbell S *et al.* (1991) Transvaginal colour Doppler assessment of the utero-placental circulation in early pregnancy. *Obstet Gynaecol* **365**: 365–9.

15 Bower S, Vyas S, Campbell S, Nicolaides K. (1992) Color flow imaging of the uterine artery in pregnancy: Normal ranges of impedance to blood flow, mean velocity and volume of flow. *Ultrasound Obstet Gynecol* **2**: 1–5.

16 Campbell S, Pearce JMF, Hackett G, Cohen-Overbeek T, Hernandex C. (1986) Qualitative assessment of uteroplacental blood flow: An early screening test for high risk pregnancies. *Obstet Gynaecol* **68**: 649–53.

17 Fleischer A, Schulman H, Farmakides G *et al.* (1986) Uterine artery Doppler velocimetry in pregnant women with hypertension. *Am J Obstet Gynecol* **154**: 806–13.

18 Steel SA, Pearce JM, Chamberlain GV. (1990) Early ultrasound screening in prediction of hypertensive disorders of pregnancy. *Lancet* **335**: 1548–52.

19 Kofinas AD, Penry M, Swain M, Hatjis CG. (1989) Effect of placental laterality on uterine artery resistance and development of pre-eclampsia and intrauterine growth retardation. *Am J Obstet Gynecol* **161**: 1536–9.

20 Schulman H, Ducey J, Farmakides G, Guzman E, Winter D, Penny B, Chi-Lee. (1987) Uterine artery Doppler velocimetry: The significance of divergent systolic/diastolic ratios. *Am J Obstet Gynecol* **157**: 1539–42.

21 Bewley S, Cooper D, Campbell S. (1991) Doppler investigation of uteroplacental blood flow in the second trimester: A screening study for pre-eclampsia and intrauterine growth retardation. *Br J Obstet Gynaecol* **98**: 871–9.

22 Harrington K, Campbell S, Bewley S, Bower S. (1991) Doppler velocimetry studies of the uterine artery in the early prediction of pre-eclampsia and intrauterine growth retardation. *Eur J Obstet Gynecol Reprod Biol* **42**: S14–20.

23 Bower S, Bewley S, Campbell S. (1993) Improved prediction of pre-eclampsia by two-stage screening of the uterine arteries using the early distolic notch and colour Doppler imaging. *Obstet Gynaecol* **82**: 78–83.

24 Harrington K, Campbell S. (1992) The prediction of pre-eclampsia using transvaginal Doppler ultrasound in early pregnancy. Proceedings of the BMUS meeting. *Br J Rad* **65**: 639.

25 Wallenburg HCS. (1986) Changes in the coagulation system and platelets-induced hypertension and pre-eclampsia. In: *Hypertension in Pregnancy*, Proceedings of the Sixteenth Study Group of the Royal College of Obstetricians and Gynaecologists, pp. 227-48. Edited by Sharp F, Symonds EM. Perinatology Press, Oxford.

26 McParland P, Pearce JM, Chamberlain GV. (1990) Doppler ultrasound and aspirin in recognition and prevention of pregnancy induced hypertension. *Lancet* **335**: 1552–4.

CHAPTER 5

The placenta and umbilical cord

Eric Jauniaux

INTRODUCTION

Colour flow imaging has revolutionized our ability to map out *in utero* the fetal and maternal components of the placental circulation.[1,2] From the second month of gestation, this new ultrasound technique allows the identification of the various branches of the main uterine arteries and the umbilical cord circulation.[3-5] As a consequence, vascular structures not seen thus far with ultrasound, especially inside the placenta, can now be seen and analysed more distinctly.[1] Since the advent of colour Doppler imaging, an increasing number of placental and cord abnormalities have been precisely diagnosed as early as the end of the first trimester of gestation. The contribution of colour Doppler imaging to the investigation of normal and abnormal placental development is illustrated in this chapter.

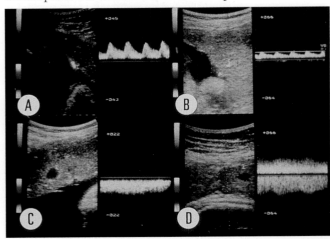

Fig. 5.1
Colour flow mapping and flow velocity waveforms of different segments of the fetal and maternal circulations. (A) Chorionic artery at 28 weeks' gestation. (B) Intraplacental arterioles at 32 weeks' gestation. (C) Venous flow pattern in periphery of a sonolucent area at 38 weeks' gestation. (D) Low resistance turbulent flow at the level of the maternal plate, under a sonolucent area, at 40 weeks' gestation.

DEVELOPMENT OF THE PLACENTAL CIRCULATION

Uteroplacental circulation

In the early weeks of human pregnancy, the spiral arteries undergo major morphological changes. They become the uteroplacental arteries which are distended low resistance channels capable of increasing the blood supply to the fetoplacental unit at term to ten times that of the non-pregnant uterus.[6]

The various branches of the uterine circulation can

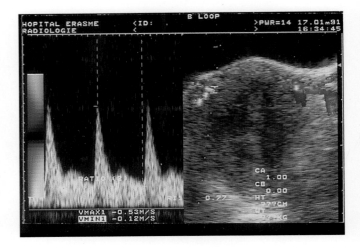

Fig. 5.2
Abdominal colour Doppler mapping and spectral analysis of blood velocity waveforms obtained from the main uterine artery at 8 weeks' gestation.

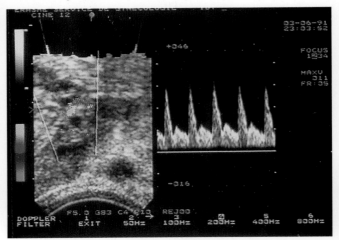

Fig. 5.3
Transvaginal colour Doppler mapping and spectral analysis of blood velocity waveforms obtained from the main uterine artery at 7 weeks' gestation. Note the well-defined protodiastolic notch.

be reliably distinguished by means of colour imaging (Fig. 5.1) and the overall Doppler features correlate well with the classic anatomic findings.[6] The two-dimensional display allows accurate placement of the Doppler gate for spectral analysis. Blood flow velocity waveforms from the main uterine arteries in normal pregnancies are characterized by a well-defined early diastolic notch (Figs 5.2 and 5.3) which disappears around 18–20 weeks of gestation.[1]

When the Doppler gate is moved towards the placental implantation site, low impedance turbulent flow, which characterizes the transformed spiral arteries, is detected (Fig. 5.4). Continuous non-pulsatile flow on colour imaging, with a venous pattern on spectral analysis, can only be detected between 12 and 14 weeks

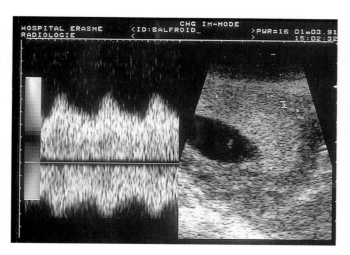

Fig. 5.4
Abdominal colour Doppler ultrasound and spectral analysis of uterplacental artery waveforms near the basal placental plate at 13 weeks' gestation showing a typical flow with an irregular and spiky outline

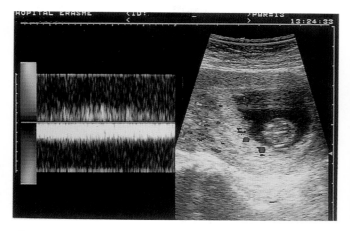

Fig. 5.5
Abdominal colour Doppler mapping and spectral analysis demonstrating continuous blood flow with a venous pattern (i.e. intervillous flow) at 13 weeks' gestation

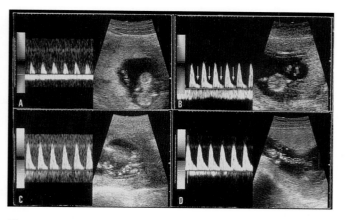

Fig. 5.6
Abdominal colour Doppler mapping and spectral analysis. (A) At 8 weeks' gestation, demonstrating regular umbilical artery waveforms with no end diastolic flow. (B) At 14 weeks (same case as in (A)) showing continuous end diastolic flow (arrows) in the umbilical artery. (C) At 13 weeks, showing continuous blood flow with a venous pattern (i.e. intervillous flow). (D) At 13 weeks, uteroplacental artery waveforms near the basal placental plate showing a typical flow with an irregular and spiky outline.

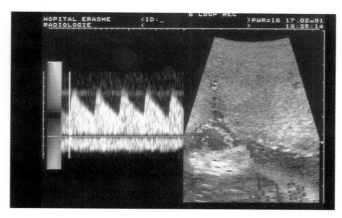

Fig. 5.7
Colour flow mapping and flow velocity waveforms of a main (stem) villous artery at 29 weeks' gestation.

of gestation when the Doppler gate is placed over intraplacental sonolucent spaces (Fig. 5.5). This flow pattern is assumed to derive from maternal intervillous blood flow which enters the intervillous space when the trophoblastic plugs no longer obliterate the utero-placental arteries.

Umbilicoplacental circulation

Umbilical flow velocity waveforms before 14 weeks of gestation are typically characterized by the absence of end diastolic velocities (Fig. 5.6). Between 12 and 14 weeks, end diastolic velocities appear. Diastolic flow is incomplete and/or inconsistently present until 14 weeks of gestation. After this, pandiastolic frequencies

are consistently present (Fig. 5.6). Intraplacental wave-forms with fetal characteristics can be identified and clearly differentiated from the beginning of the second trimester (Fig. 5.7).

The appearance of end diastolic frequencies in the umbilical circulation coincides with an abrupt and significant increase in uterine artery peak systolic velocity together with the presence of continuous intervillous flow within the whole placental mass.[7] The establishment of the intervillous circulation may be associated with changes in the pressure gradient due to the expansion of the intervillous space and/or with modification in blood gases and metabolite concentrations which in turn may explain the rapid appearance of end diastolic frequencies in the umbilical circulation.[2]

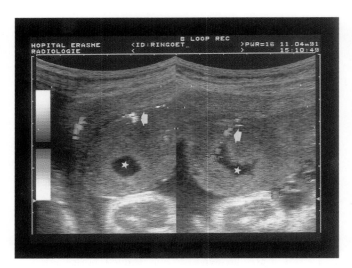

Fig. 5.8
Colour flow mapping of the placenta at 32 weeks' gestation showing the terminal part of a uteroplacental vessel (arrow) entering a placental lake (star)

Placental anatomy and abnormalities

The gross anatomy of the human placenta is basically the anatomy of its fetal circulation with connective tissue support and trophoblastic covering.[6] The maternal tissues contribute little to the architecture of the definitive placenta. At the end of the first trimester, the placenta can be clearly separated into three basic structures: the chorionic or fetal plate, the placental villous tissue or substance and the basal or maternal plate.[6]

Circulation of maternal blood through the intervillous chamber is a dynamic process that requires a continuous adaptation of the individual cotyledon to the flow offered to it by the corresponding uteroplacental artery. Compromises in placental circulatory homoeostasis are associated with significant fetal complications resulting from disruption of an adequate supply of oxygen and nutrients.

Sonolucent areas within the placenta vary from small hypoechoic spaces to large sonolucent spaces, also called 'maternal lakes', and are secondary to the dispersion of the free-floating terminal villi by maternal arterial jets of blood entering the intervillous space (Fig. 5.8). Maternal lakes correspond to a non-pathologic variation of the placental structure, which occurs early in pregnancy.[8]

Most placental vascular and non-vascular lesions can be diagnosed prenatally by ultrasound.[8,9] The localization of the lesion, its size and its echogenicity on serial ultrasound examinations are critical for prenatal recognition of the different placental lesions (Table 5.1).

Table 5.1 Pathologic classification, sonographic features and the most common clinical complications of the principal placental abnormalities.

Pathologic classification	Sonographic features	Location	Associated complications
Vascular lesions			
Thrombosis	Sonolucent → hyperechoic Turbulent BF	Intervillous Subchorial	Isoimmunization
Infarcts	Hyperechoic → isoechoic Irregular shape and no BF	Maternal plate	PIH and/or IUGR
Haematomas	Hyperechoic → hypoechoic → sonolucent and no BF	Subamniotic Retroplacental	IUGR PIH
Fibrin	Hyperechoic and no BF	Diffuse	IUGR
Non-trophoblastic tumours			
Chorioangioma	Hypoechoic → hypoechoic Round and encapsulated and BF with fetal features	Fetal plate or intraplacental	Polyhydramnios NIHF-IUGR
Mesenchymal hyperplasia	Multiple small hypoechoic spaces often containing BF	Diffuse in normal placenta	Giant placenta
Trophoblastic tumours			
Classic mole	Snowstorm appearance with no fetus and no BF	Diffuse	Vaginal bleeding, severe vomiting, PIH, ovarian cysts
Triploidy	Swiss cheese appearance with no BF with a fetus	Diffuse	IUGR, PIH, hydramnios
Abnormalities of placentation			
Placenta circumvallate	Mammelonnated fetal plate and marginal haematoma	Placental margin	PROM, premature labour
Placenta accreta	No placental-uterine interface and dilated vessels	Maternal plate	Vaginal bleeding, uterine rupture
Placenta membranacea	Uterine cavity covered with placental tissue	Continuous placenta	Vaginal bleeding, premature labour

IUGR = intrauterine growth retardation; PROM = premature rupture of membranes; PIH = pregnancy-induced hypertension; NIHF = non-immune hydrops fetalis; BF = blood flow (on colour mapping)

A sonographic classification of the placental lesions based on their location, size, echogenicity and number has been recently proposed.[9] Only a few placental abnormalities have thus far been investigated by means of colour Doppler imaging.

Vascular lesions

Placental thromboses are the result of focal coagulation of blood in the intervillous spaces and occur more frequently in pregnancies complicated by rhesus isoimmunization.[8] Abnormal haemodynamic flow in the

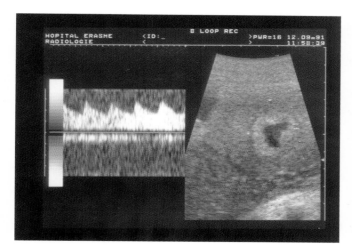

Fig. 5.9
Colour flow mapping and flow velocity waveforms of a main (stem) villous artery surrounding an intervillous thrombosis. No flow is detected inside the lesion which is surrounded by a ring of degenerative hyperechogenic villi.

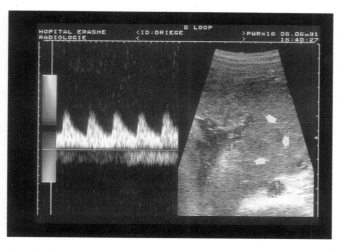

Fig. 5.10
Heterogenous intraplacental mass (arrow), under the cord insertion at 25 weeks' gestation corresponding to a cellular chorioangioma after delivery. Flow velocity waveforms at the periphery of the tumour were of fetal origin.

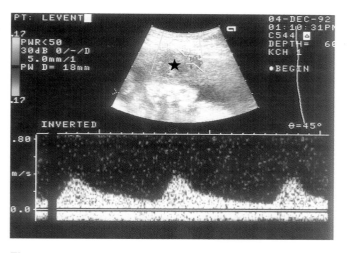

Fig. 5.11
Colour flow mapping and flow velocity waveforms of a mass (star) located at the placental edge. All signals showed maternal characteristics suggesting the diagnosis of uterine myoma.

intervillous space may result from the failure of the cotyledon to expand in response to the increasing flow of the corresponding uteroplacental artery and compression of the surrounding villi which gradually become atrophied as fibrin is laid down in the periphery.[8,9] This process causes a progressive increase in the echogenicity of the lesion (Fig. 5.9). Finally the maternal blood coagulates in the placental tissue, focally obliterating the intervillous circulation.

Placental infarcts are the result of arteriolar obstruction of the uteroplacental artery leading to focal degeneration of the overlying villous tissue.[8,9] The incidence of placental infarction is significantly increased in pregnancies complicated by pre-eclampsia or essential hypertension and is directly related to the severity of the disease. Infarcts involving more than 10% of the placental parenchyma are associated with an increase in perinatal mortality and intrauterine growth retardation. Sonographically, they appear as large intraplacental areas, irregular and hyperechoic in the acute stage and isoechoic in the more advanced stages. Placental infarcts are usually located near the basal plate and contain no blood flow from either the maternal or fetal circulation.

Placental tumours

Chorioangiomas are usually single, encapsulated, small, round lesions located within the placental mass.[9] Chorioangiomas are associated with an increased incidence of polyhydramnios and fetal growth retardation. Large tumours are sometimes complicated by fetal cardiac failure with hydrops due to the shunting of blood through the tumour. The fetal risk probably depends more on the proportion of angiomatous to myxoid tissue inside the tumour than on its exact size. With ultrasound, chorioangiomas appear as well circumscribed lesions with a different echogenicity from the rest of the placental tissue (Fig. 5.10). They often protrude into the amniotic cavity. The echogenicity varies according to the degree of degenerative changes present in the tumour.[9] The vascular nature of the tumour can easily be evaluated *in utero* with colour Doppler imaging.[1]

Knowledge of the normal fetal and placental Doppler waveform characteristics is important if the differential diagnosis of placental and other intrauterine abnormalities is to be helped by Doppler ultrasound.[1] For example, in cases of an undetermined placental mass, demonstration of fetal waveforms strongly suggests chorioangioma (Fig. 5.10), whereas maternal waveforms favour the diagnosis of uterine myoma (Fig. 5.11).

Hydatidiform moles are classified into two distinct entities, i.e. complete and partial mole.[9] Complete hydatidiform moles are characterized by generalized swelling of the villous tissue, trophoblastic hyperplasia and no embryonic or fetal tissue. Complete moles are almost always diploid with a 46,XX chromosomal constitution in more than 90% of cases.

Partial hydatidiform moles are characterized by focal swelling of the villous tissue, focal trophoblastic hyperplasia and embryonic or fetal tissue. The most common karyotype found in these cases is triploidy. Following uterine evacuation, persistent gestational trophoblastic disease occurs in about 15–20% of patients with complete mole and in about 4–5% of patients with partial mole.[10] Colour Doppler imaging has an important role to play in the early and non-invasive diagnosis and treatment of this complication.[11, 12]

Abnormality of placentation

Placenta accreta is defined as a placenta with abnormal adherence to the uterine wall, with either partial or complete invasion into the myometrium.[13, 14] This abnormality is characterized by myometrial invasion by the villi and occurs when the decidua basalis is partially or completely absent. According to the degree of myometrial invasion, this condition is subdivided into placenta accreta vera when the villi are simply attached to the myometrium, placenta increta when the villi deeply invade the myometrium, and placenta percreta when the villi penetrate the entire thickness of the uterine wall.

All conditions or procedures which affect the integrity of the uterine wall, e.g. caesarean section and other uterine surgery, curettage, sepsis or fibroids, are predisposing factors for abnormal villous penetration. In many patients there is a combination of these aetiological factors: the association of a prior uterine scar and low placental insertion is a particular risk. Pregnancies affected by placenta accreta have a high maternal and fetal mortality due to antepartum or postpartum bleeding, uterine rupture and uterine inversion. On ultrasound, the decidual interface between placenta and myometrium (clear space) is absent at the level of the abnormal villous penetration and multiple dilated blood vessels are present beneath the placental tissue.[13, 14] Prenatal diagnosis of this condition may allow the obstetrician to demarcate the areas of the placenta that require resection before surgery (Fig. 5.12).

UMBILICAL CORD ANATOMY AND ABNORMALITIES

The anatomy of the umbilical cord can be visualized around 20 week' gestation by grey scale imaging, but a precise diagnosis of a particular cord abnormality may be difficult and time consuming. At the end of the second or during the third trimester, the umbilical cord anatomy can be examined in detail with less difficulty. However, various factors such as oligohydramnios or

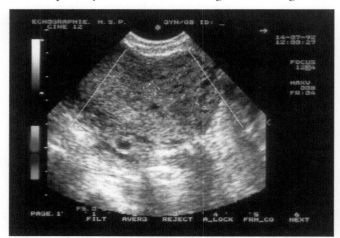

Fig. 5.12
Colour flow mapping of the uterine wall in a patient presenting with post partum bleeding showing multiple dilated blood vessels deep inside the uterine myometrium. Pathological investigation of the hysterectomy specimen demonstrated placenta increta (courtesy of Dr. M van Rysselberge).

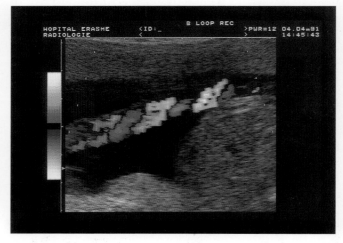

Fig. 5.13
Longitudinal colour scan at 22 weeks' gestation showing the normal anatomy of the umbilical cord with two arteries and one vein

multiple loops of cord can make accurate visualization of the cord vessels impossible, even near term.

Colour Doppler imaging has proved to be an efficient tool for the early and accurate diagnosis of most cord abnormalities. It is also of clinical value in assisting with invasive procedures such as amniocentesis or cordocentesis.[8, 14, 15]

Abnormal cord insertion

The umbilical arteries branch off the hypogastric arteries, course lateral to the bladder onto the anterior abdominal wall and then through the umbilical cord to the placenta (Figs 5.13–5.15). Marginal and markedly eccentric placental insertions of the cord are not associated with an excess of pregnancy complications but may indicate a malrotation of the blastocyst at implantation, as suggested by an increased incidence of this anomaly in IVF pregnancies.[14] Placenta velamentosa is a well defined pathologic entity with an incidence of 1%.[14]

From a clinical point of view, attachment of the cord to the extraplacental membranes is important because of the risk of severe fatal haemorrhage during labour.[16, 17] Antenatal diagnosis of attachment of the cord to the membranes rather than the placental mass can be diagnosed before labour by means of colour imaging (Fig. 5.16).

Abnormal number of vessels

The absence of one umbilical artery is amongst the most common congenital fetal malformations with an incidence of approximately 1% of all deliveries.[18] Major fetal anatomic defects are largely responsible for the high fetal and neonatal loss from this pathology. Fetal malformations are present in about 50% of the cases of single umbilical artery and can affect any organ system (Table 5.2). The incidence of intrauterine growth retardation is significantly elevated among fetuses with only one umbilical artery and may be present without other congenital anomalies in 15–20% of cases.[18] Colour imaging has an important role to play in the early and accurate diagnosis of a single umbilical artery (Fig. 5.17).

During the second month of fetal development, the right umbilical vein regresses and the left umbilical vein and the two umbilical arteries become the vessels found in the normal cord. The persistence of a right umbili-

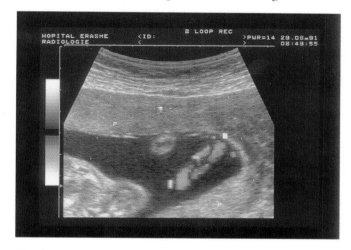

Fig. 5.15
Colour flow mapping of the placental insertion of the umbilical cord at 28 weeks. Note that the placenta is bilobate. The placental lobes are connected by a thin bridge of placental tissue where the cord is inserted (square).

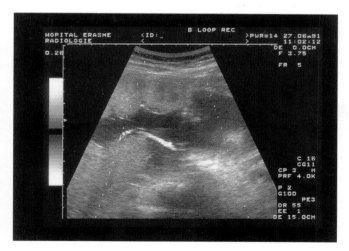

Fig. 5.16
Colour flow mapping of the placental insertion of the umbilical cord at 34 weeks. The umbilical vessels split before reaching the fetal plate of the placenta suggesting a velamentous insertion of the cord.

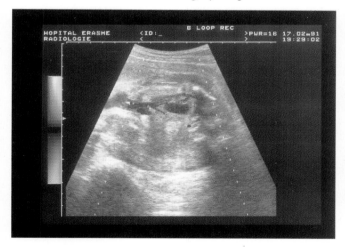

Fig. 5.14
Colour flow mapping of the fetal pelvis at 22 weeks showing the origin of the umbilical arteries

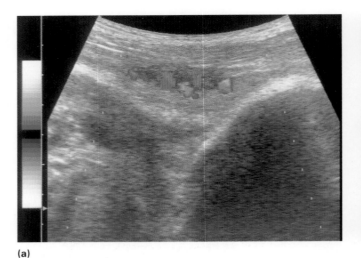

(a)

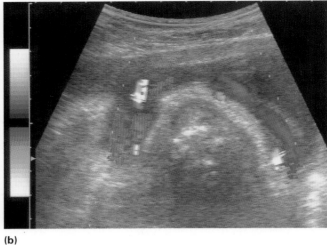

(b)

Fig. 5.17
Longitudinal (a) and traverse (b) colour imaging of the fetal neck region at 36 weeks' gestation showing features suggesting a nuchal cord

cal vein is an uncommon finding which can be associated with occasionally lethal fetal malformations.[19] This cord abnormality is easily recognized during the second trimester and is an indication for more in-depth scanning of the fetus.

Table 5.2 Comparison of prenatal sonographic features and postnatal findings in a series of 80 cases of SUA (Modified from reference 18).

Comparative Data (n = 80)	Sonographic features	Postnatal findings
Number of fetuses with associated malformation(s)	21 (26.6%)	34 (42.5%)
Total IUGR	28.3%	36.4%
Isolated IUGR	15%	20%
Distribution of the different associated fetal malformations		
• Musculoskeletel system	15 (28.8%)	32 (32%)
• Urogenital system	11 (21.1%)	20 (20%)
• Gastrointestinal system	5 (5.8%)	11 (11%)
• Central nervous system	12 (23.1%)	11 (11%)
• Integument	3 (5.8%)	9 (9%)
• Cardiovascular system	4 (7.7%)	8 (8%)
• Respiratory system	4 (7.7%)	6 (6%)
• Miscellaneous	– (0%)	3 (3%)
Total	52 (100%)	100 (100%)

IUGR = intrauterine growth retardation

Looping and prolapse of the cord

Looping of the cord may occur around the fetal neck, body or shoulder and can be accurately diagnosed by colour imaging (Fig. 5.17). The overall sensitivity of colour imaging (78.9%) in detecting nuchal cord prenatally is significantly higher than that of grey scale imaging (33.3%). Although single looping of the cord around the neck is an uncommon cause of fetal death, umbilical cord problems in monoamniotic twins con-

tribute to the high mortality rate.[14] The clinical usefulness of systematic identification *in utero* of nuchal cord in pregnancies presenting with a normal fetus in the vertex position is limited but can be of great value in the management of breech and twin gestations and of chronically growth retarded fetuses.[20]

Prolapse of the umbilical cord is an obstetric emergency characterized by protrusion of the umbilical cord through the cervix into the vagina.[14] Cord prolapse is more likely to occur during premature labour, with long umbilical cords, an unengaged presenting part or in pregnancies complicated by polyhydramnios.[14] Sonography can easily demonstrate, in the lower segment, fine parallel linear echoes corresponding to the cord, below the presenting part.

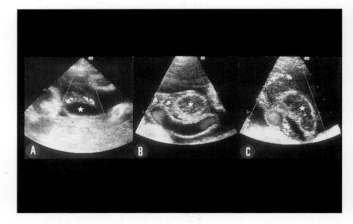

Fig. 5.20
Colour flow mapping of the fetal insertion of the umbilical cord. (A) At 18 weeks showing a hypoechoic cavity (star) corresponding to a cord pseudocyst. B and C at 32 weeks, showing a small omphalocele (star) above dilated umbilical vein.

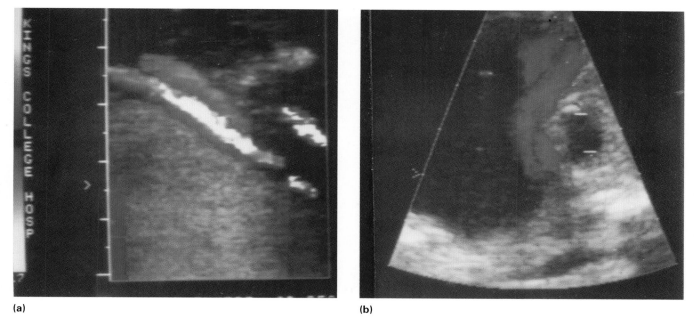

Fig. 5.18
Colour flow image of single umbilical artery cord. (a) At 18 weeks, associated with multiple fetal malformations and oligohydramnios (b) (reproduced from reference 15).

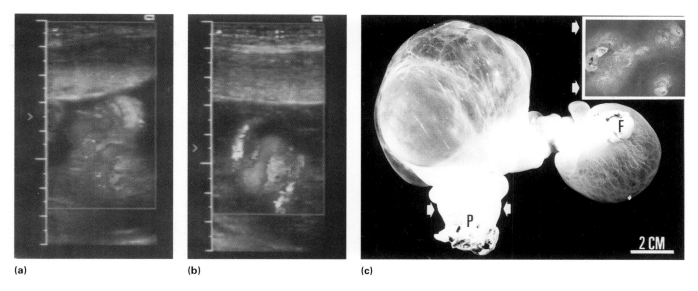

Fig. 5.19
Colour flow image of a cord tumour at 36 weeks' gestation showing an abnormal vascular pattern at the placental insertion (a) and the tumoral tissue, which is hyperechogenic compared to the Wharton's jelly and surrounds the umbilical vein (b) (reproduced from reference 15). (c) View of the cord after delivery demonstrating two areas of oedema, corresponding to pseudocysts. The tumour starts near the placental insertion (P) and ends 2 cm from the fetal umbilici (F). The tumour is made of small capillary vessels proliferating around the main umbilical vessels (insert).

Umbilical cord tumours and vascular lesions

From a pathological point of view, primary cord tumours can be divided into angiomyxomas or haemangiomas derived from embryonic vessels, teratomas derived from germ cells and vestigial cysts derived from remnants of the allantois or the omphalomesenteric duct.[14] A cord angiomyxoma appears sonographically as a heterogeneous mass presenting a strong echogenic area, embedding the umbilical vessels (Fig. 5.19) and surrounded by large echopoor areas.[15] The prenatal diagnosis of cord teratomas has never been reported but

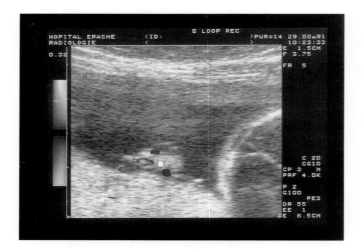

Fig. 5.21
Intense echogenic lesion appearing inside the umbilical cord at the site of umbilical puncture for fetal transfusion and associated with short term disappearance of end diastolic flow in the umbilical artery

this type of tumour should be mainly composed of dense tissue.[14] Conversely, vestigial cysts appear sonographically as a single fluid-filled mass. Vestigial cysts and pseudocysts can sometimes be associated with small abdominal wall defects (Fig. 5.20) and a precise early prenatal diagnosis can be more difficult to establish.[21]

Several conditions causing simple or complex multi-cystic cord masses can mimic a tumour on ultrasound imaging. These conditions include cord haematomas, ectasia of the umbilical vein, pseudocysts and true knots.[14, 22] Prenatal identification of a cord haematoma is of particular interest as it may be induced by an accidental laceration of umbilical cord vessels during an invasive procedure.[23] The end result of a cord haematoma may range from complete occlusion of the cord vessels with inevitable fetal death to varying degrees of fetal distress, either acute or chronic. Ultrasound can readily detect the development of a potentially harmful haematoma at the site of puncture and Doppler velocimetry may indicate tamponade of the umbilical cord vessels (Fig. 5.21).

REFERENCES

1 Jauniaux E, Jurkovic D, Campbell S, Kurjak A, Hustin J. (1991) Investigation of placental circulations by colour Doppler ultrasound. *Am J Obstet Gynecol* **164**: 486–8.

2 Jauniaux E, Jurkovic D, Campbell S. (1991) In vivo investigations of the anatomy and the physiology of early human placental circulations. *Ultrasound Obstet Gynecol* **1**: 435–45.

3 Jurkovic D, Jauniaux E, Kurjak A, Hustin J, Campbell S, Nicolaides KH. (1991) Transvaginal colour Doppler assessment of utero-placental circulation in early pregnancy. *Obstet Gynaecol* **77**: 365–9.

4 Jaffe R, Warsof SL. (1991) Transvaginal color Doppler imaging in the assessment of uteroplacental blood flow in the normal first-trimester pregnancy. *Am J Obstet Gynecol* **164**: 781–5.

5 Jurkovic D, Jauniaux E, Campbell S. (1992) Doppler ultrasound investigations of pelvic circulation during the menstrual cycle and early pregnancy. In: *The First Twelve Weeks of Gestation*, pp. 78–96. Edited by Barnea E, Hustin J, Jauniaux E. Springer-Verlag, Heidelberg.

6 Ramsey EM, Donner NW. (1980) *Placental Vasculature and Circulation*. Georg Thieme, Stuttgart.

7 Jauniaux E, Jurkovic D, Campbell S, Hustin J. (1992) Doppler ultrasonographic features of the developing placental circulations: Correlation with anatomic findings. *Am J Obstet Gynecol* **166**: 585–7.

8 Jauniaux E, Campbell S. (1992) Perinatal assessment of placental and cord abnormalities. In: *Ultrasound in obstetrics and gynaecology*, pp. 327–43. Edited by Chervenak FA, Isaacson G, Campbell S. Little, Brown and Company, Boston.

9 Jauniaux E, Campbell S. (1990) Sonographic assessment of placental abnormalities. *Am J Obstet Gynecol* **163**: 1650–8.

10 Flam F, Lindholm H, Bui TH, Lundstrom-Lindstedt V. (1991) Colour Doppler studies in trophoblastic tumors. *Ultrasound Obstet Gynecol* **1**: 349–52.

11 Long MG, Boultbee JE, Langley R, Newlands ES, Begent RHJ, Bagshawe KD. (1992) Doppler assessment of the uterine circulation and the clinical behaviour of gestational trophoblastic tumours requiring chemotherapy. *Br J Cancer* **66**: 883–7.

12 Chou MM, Ho ESC, Lu F, Lee YH. (1992) Prenatal diagnosis of placenta previa/accreta with colour Doppler ultrasound. *Ultrasound Obstet Gynecol* **2**: 293–6.

13 Rosemond RL, Kepple DM. (1992) Transvaginal colour Doppler in the prenatal diagnosis of placenta accreta. *Obstet Gynaecol* **80**: 508–9.

14 Jauniaux E, Campbell S. (1993) Ultrasonographic diagnosis of placental and cord abnormalities. In: *Clinical Ultrasound: A Comprehensive Text, Vol III*: 435–62. Edited by Meire H, Cosgrove D, Dewbury K. Churchill Livingstone, London.

15 Jauniaux E, Campbell S, Vyas S. (1989) The use of color Doppler imaging for prenatal diagnosis of umbilical cord anomalies: Report of three cases. *Am J Obstet Gynecol* **161**: 1195–7.

16 Nelson LH, Melone PJ, King M. (1990) Diagnosis of vasa previa with transvaginal and colour flow Doppler ultrasound. *Obstet Gynaecol* **76**: 506–9.

17 Harding JA, Lewis DF, Major CA, Crade M, Patel J, Nageotte MP. (1990) Color flow Doppler: A useful instrument in the diagnosis of vasa previa. *Am J Obstet Gynecol* **163**: 1566–8.

18 Jauniaux E, De Munter C, Pardou A, Elkhazen N, Rodesch F, Wilkin P. (1989) Evaluation échographique du syndrôme de l'artère ombilicale unique: Une série de 80 cas. *J Gynécol Obstet Biol Reprod* **18**: 341–8.

19 Jeanty P. (1990) Persistent right umbilical vein: An ominous prenatal finding. *Radiology* **177**: 735–8.

20 Jauniaux E, Mawissa C, Peellaerts C, Rodesch F. (1992) Nuchal cord in normal third trimester pregnancy: A colour Doppler imaging study. *Ultrasound Obstet Gynecol* **2**: 417–19.

21 Jauniaux E, Jurkovic D, Campbell S. (1991) Sonographic features of an umbilical cord abnormality combining a cord pseudocyst and a small omphalocele. *Eur J Obstet Gynecol Reprod Biol* **38**: 245–8.

22 Rizzo G, Arduini D. (1992) Prenatal diagnosis of an intra-abdominal ectasia of the umbilical vein with colour Doppler ultrasonography. *Ultrasound Obstet Gynecol* **2**: 55–7.

23 Jauniaux E, Nicolaides KH, Campbell S, Hustin J. (1990) Hematoma of the umbilical cord secondary to cordocentesis for intrauterine fetal transfusion. *Prenat Diagn* **10**: 477–8.

CHAPTER 6

The fetal arterial circulation

Stuart Campbell, Kevin Harrington and Kurt Hecher

INTRODUCTION

Understanding circulatory changes in health and disease is one of the cornerstones of medical practice, with every medical student learning to appreciate the importance of taking a pulse and blood pressure reading as one of the first steps in any physical examination. Prior to the introduction of Doppler ultrasound we could listen for the fetal heart, and more recently with the introduction of fetal heart rate monitors, appreciate alterations in the variability of the fetal heart rate pattern, but we were unable to examine the dynamics of the fetal circulation in any detail. Although we still cannot measure blood pressure directly in the fetus, Doppler ultrasound allows non-invasive assessment of fetal haemodynamics.

Doppler investigation of the umbilical artery provides information on perfusion of the fetoplacental circulation whilst Doppler studies of selected fetal organs are valuable in detecting the haemodynamic rearrangements that occur in response to fetal hypoxia and anaemia. Animal studies have demonstrated that during hypoxia there is a preferential perfusion of the fetal brain, heart and adrenals at the expense of the carcass, gut and kidneys; this adaptation is termed the brain-sparing effect.[1] Ultrasound biometric measurements of the human fetus have demonstrated an alteration in the head:abdomen circumference ratio in favour of head growth in the small for gestational age (SGA) fetus that is growth retarded[2] and more recently, Doppler ultrasound has enabled the non-invasive confirmation of the brain-sparing effect in human fetuses.[3] This chapter demonstrates how fetal Doppler waveforms are obtained from the arterial circulation, and summarizes the changes with advancing gestation in fetal Doppler parameters in the appropriately grown fetus. This introduces the potential use of fetal Doppler ultrasound of the arterial circulation in the management of the at risk fetus. This theme is expanded upon in the Chapter 'The fetal haemodynamic response to hypoxia'.

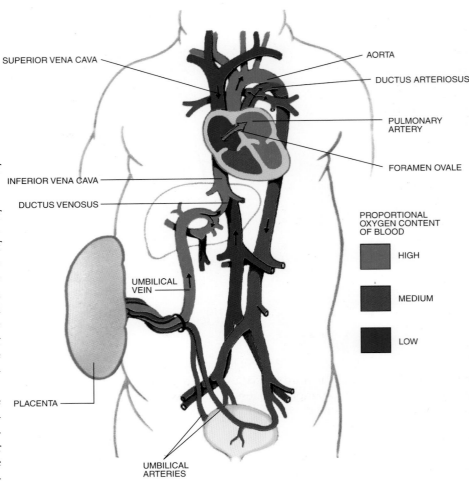

Fig. 6.1
Diagrammatic representation of fetal circulation.

OBTAINING DOPPLER SIGNALS FROM THE FETAL ARTERIAL CIRCULATION

The fetal arterial circulation differs from the neonatal circulation in two respects: blood from the right side of the heart is shunted, via the foramen ovale and ductus arteriosus to the left side of the heart and aorta respectively, bypassing the lungs (Fig. 6.1). Also about 50% of the blood flow through the aorta passes back to the placenta via the umbilical arteries.

The umbilical arteries

Flow velocity waveforms (FVW) from the umbilical artery (UA) can be easily obtained using CW or pulsed wave Doppler ultrasound,[4] and the finding of elevated

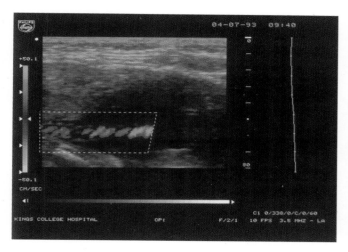

Fig. 6.2

Helical pattern of umbilical vessels illustrated with colour velocity imaging (see Fig. 6.1). Colour is not usually necessary to identify the cord. It can be useful when the cord insertion is posterior, or when there is reduced amniotic fluid.

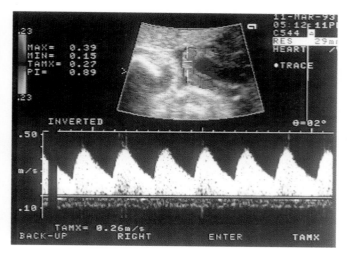

Fig. 6.3

A normal umbilical artery (UA) flow velocity waveform from the second half of pregnancy with abundant diastolic flow. It is possible to measure changes in resistance using a calculated index of resistance, e.g. the pulsatility index, or by noting the presence or absence of diastolic flow.

umbilical artery resistance is consistently associated with a poor perinatal outcome.[5] If using CW Doppler, the position of the umbilical cord can be initially identified with real-time ultrasound, before obtaining the FVW. This is usually a simple process, except when there is oligohydramnios, a posterior placenta, or the fetal spine is anterior. With colour flow/velocity imaging it is possible to appreciate the helical pattern of the umbilical vessels (Fig. 6.2). It is difficult to mistake the umbilical artery FVW because of the characteristic saw-tooth appearance of arterial flow in one direction and continuous umbilical venous blood flow in the other (Fig. 6.3). For this reason colour flow is not usually needed.

Doppler signals can be acquired from different points in the cord, at the umbilical insertion, the placental insertion, or anywhere along the cord (Fig. 6.4). Although the indices of resistance change according to the location along the cord, the differences are not usually sufficient to alter the interpretation of the result.[6] When obtaining a FVW from the umbilical arteries, and indeed from anywhere in the fetal circulation, it is important to ensure that the fetus is not breathing, as this can dramatically alter the value obtained (Fig. 6.5). In practice we usually obtain FVWs from a mid point in the cord, or near the placental insertion.

Much of the interpretation of fetal Doppler rests on a comparison of the distribution of blood flow to the

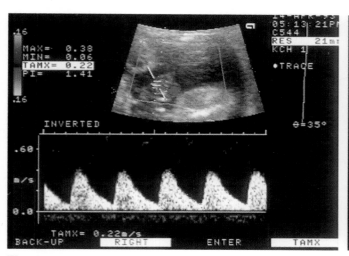

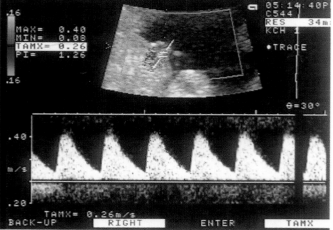

Fig. 6.4

Flow velocity waveforms obtained from the same umbilical artery, at the umbilical insertion into the anterior abdominal wall, where resistance is marginally greater than at the placental insertion of the umbilical cord.

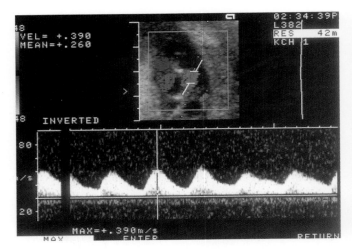

Fig. 6.5
Fetal breathing movements will alter the values obtained from
the flow velocity waveform. It is important to wait until FBM
have stopped before taking a measurement.

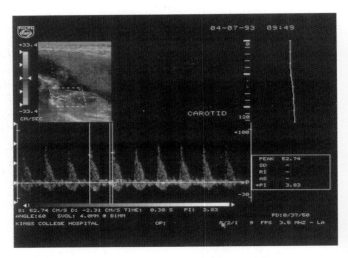

Fig. 6.6
The common carotid artery arising from the aorta. Before the
introduction of colour Doppler the carotid artery was used to
assess changes in flow to the fetal brain. Low resistance in this
vessel implies redistribution to the fetal brain, indicating
hypoxia. With the introduction of CDI, the middle cerebral artery
has become more popular for this purpose.

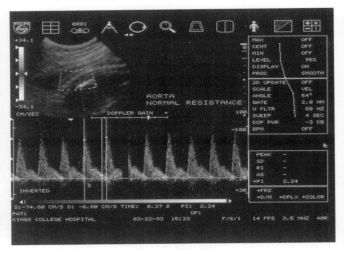

Fig. 6.7
FVWs obtained from the abdominal aorta. The abdominal aorta
resembles a FVW from one of the umbilical arteries. The
thoracic aorta reflects changes in cardiac function as well as
distal changes in the circulation of the fetus and placenta.

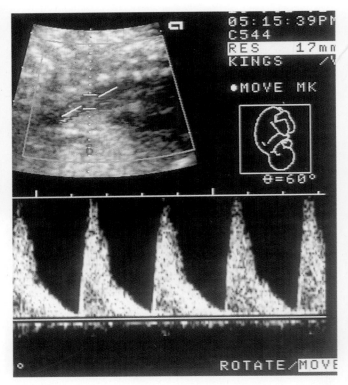

Fig. 6.8
The angle of insonation of a vessel should be no greater than 60°
if velocity measurements are being calculated. Although indices
of resistance should not be altered by the angle of insonation, an
acute angle will predispose to errors of interpretation, and will
cause problems especially for the qualitative assessment of the
flow velocity waveform. This is particularly important when
examining the thoracic aorta, as there is often a small amount of
end diastolic flow present in the normal fetus.

head compared to the rest of the body. It is important
therefore to be able to obtain reproducible signals from
the aorta and vessels to the head. The introduction of
pulsed wave Doppler ultrasound,[7] and more recently
colour flow imaging, has allowed us to study the fetal
circulation in greater detail (Fig. 6.6).[8, 9]

Aorta and carotid arteries

A longitudinal view of the fetus is necessary to locate
the common carotid artery as it arises from the aorta.
The fetal aorta is found in the same plane as the carotid

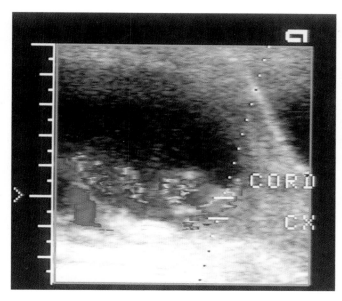

Fig. 6.9
A colour image of a vasia previa. The placenta was sited anteriorly but the cord insertion was on the posterior wall of the uterus. Colour flow imaging identified the umbilical artery as it crossed the cervix.

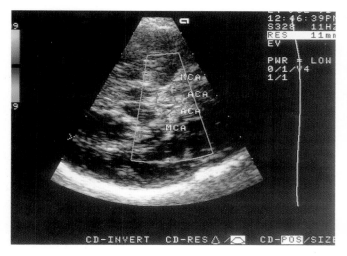

Fig. 6.10
The middle cerebral artery branching from the circle of Willis can be easily identified with colour Doppler imaging

(Figs 6.7 and 6.8). It can be difficult to secure a good angle of insonation for the aorta, as the longitudinal fetal position is parallel to the transducer. By tilting the transducer, an angle of 60° or less can be created (Fig. 6.9). Acquiring optimum signals from these vessels requires practice. It is essential to start in the right plane and practice until consistent results are obtained.

Middle cerebral arteries

The common carotid artery supplies the tissues of the head and neck in addition to the brain, but the cerebral

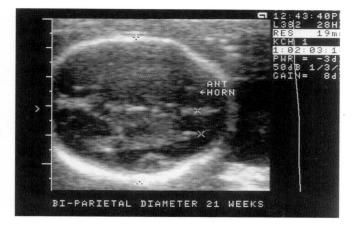

Fig. 6.11
Transverse B-mode image of the fetal head at the level of the parietal bones. This image is familiar to obstetric sonographers as the position for measuring the biparietal diameter (BPD).

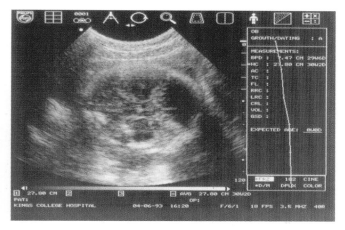

Fig. 6.12
After obtaining the BPD inmage, by moving, in the same plane, to the base of the brain, the lesser wing of the sphenoid bone is seen

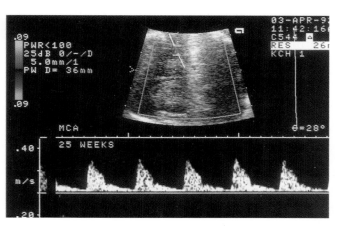

Fig. 6.13
A normal image of the middle cerebral artery waveform in the second trimester. There is a fall in resistance in the third trimester. With hypoxia the fall in resistance is more profound.

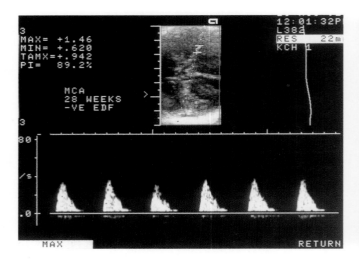

Fig. 6.14
If too much pressure is applied when trying to obtain a FVW
from the MCA, absent EDF can be seen which reappears when
pressure is eased. It is important to ensure that a true
representation of cerebral flow is obtained.

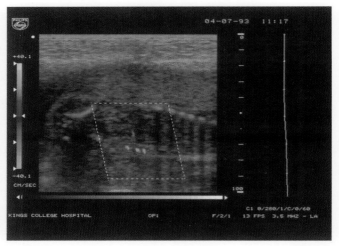

Fig. 6.16
The renal artery is easily identified with colour Doppler
imaging. A reduction in amniotic fluid volume is associated
with uteroplacental insufficiency. Changes in renal blood flow
may help in identifying the different causes of oligohydramnios.

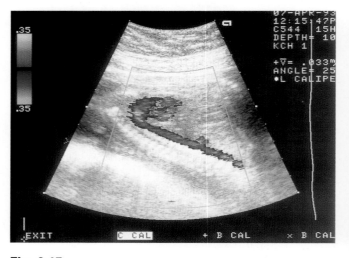

Fig. 6.15
Colour flow image of the fetal aorta. About 50% of the blood
flow through the abdominal aorta passes through the umbilical
arteries and back to the placenta. The remainder supplies the
pelvis and lower limbs via the iliac arteries.

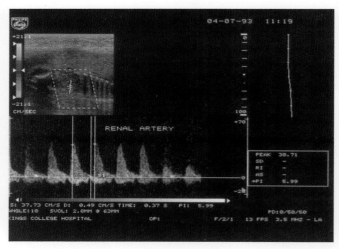

Fig. 6.17
The FVW of the renal artery usually shows a high resistance
pattern, often with absent end diastolic frequencies. This limits
the ability of the renal artery to help in the prediction or
assessment of reduced urine output. Renal artery flow may be
of more use where there is an increase in urine output, e.g. fetal
anaemia.

circulation is likely to give more precise information
about changes within the fetal brain itself. With colour
flow imaging it is possible to identify the individual
cerebral arteries (Fig. 6.10).[10] The first step in obtaining signals from the MCA is to secure an image of the
head suitable for obtaining a measurement of the
biparietal diameter (Fig. 6.11). Remaining in the same
plane, move to the base of the brain until the sphenoid bones are seen (Fig. 6.12). The MCA conveniently courses along the greater wing of the sphenoid
bone, and can readily be seen when colour Doppler is
applied (Fig. 6.13). Care must be taken to ensure that

compression by the transducer does not alter the values
obtained (Fig. 6.14).[11]

Renal arteries

The renal artery arises at a 90° angle to the aorta, and is
best seen when the abdominal aorta is visualized in a
longitudinal view, with the bifurcation into the iliac
arteries seen in the same image as the aorta (Fig. 6.15).
With colour flow imaging to assist in identifying the

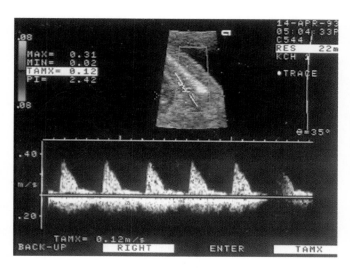

Fig. 6.18

The external iliac artery becomes the femoral artery as it passes into the leg. Resistance in the femoral artery is typically elevated in the presence of fetal acidaemia, the 'hindquarter reflex'. The aorta is at present the preferred vessel for assesing the fetal response to acidaemia.

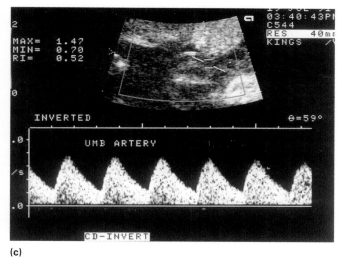

(c)

Fig. 6.19

End diastolic frequencies are usually present in the umbilical arteries by 16 weeks. The amount of end diastolic frequencies increases with gestation. Shown here are three umbilical artery waveforms, taken at 13(a), 25(b), and 35(c) weeks.

renal artery and vein (Fig. 6.16), a renal artery FVW can be obtained (Fig. 6.17). As there is a greater amount of fetal trunk movement compared to head movement, obtaining reliable signals from the renal arteries can take longer than from the MCA. Colour flow imaging allows the examination of many other arteries in the fetus, although a clinical role for these vessels has as yet not been established (Fig. 6.18).

PHYSIOLOGICAL CHANGES IN THE UMBILICAL AND ARTERIAL FETAL CIRCULATION DURING PREGNANCY

Volume flow studies of the fetal circulation

Our understanding of physiological and pathophysiological change in fetal haemodynamics would ideally be through the measurement of absolute volume flow in a particular vessel. Volume flow (Q) is calculated from the product of time averaged mean velocity (TAV) and the cross-sectional area of the vessel lumen (πr^2). Current methods of measuring volume flow using real-time and Doppler ultrasound images are limited by the large degree of error that occurs with these calculations.[12] The main sources of error are measurement of the vessel diameter, especially if the vessel is of small calibre, and in the error in estimating fetal weight when correlating volume flow by weight.[13] In a controlled setting the sources of error can be minimized and variations in measurement kept to about 10%.[14] Although

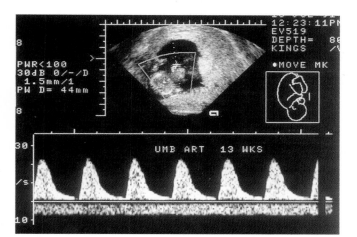

Fig. 6.19 (a)

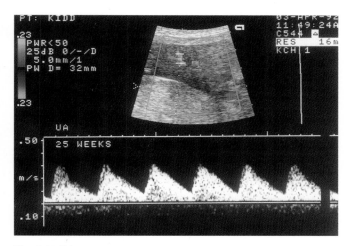

Fig. 6.18 (b)

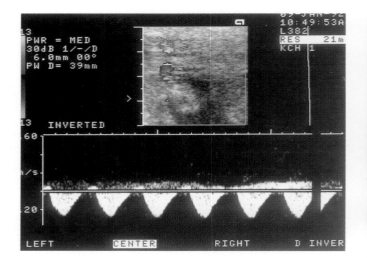

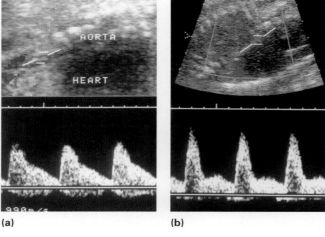

(a)

(b)

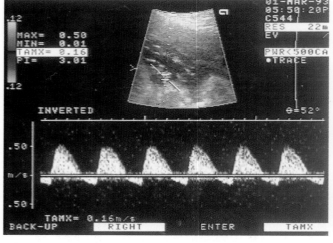

(b)

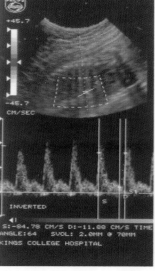

(c)

Fig. 6.20
Absent (a) or reversed end diastolic frequencies (b) in the umbilical arteries are an ominous sign in the second half of pregnancy. It is necessary to look at the fetal circulation to ascertain its response to the reduced placental supply.

Fig. 6.21
Unlike the umbilical artery, end diastolic frequencies in the aorta remain relatively constant in the second half of pregnancy. This highlights the difference in looking at the fetal and umbilical circulation, as it is often incorrectly claimed that changes in the aorta directly reflect changes in the umbilical arteries. Although much of the aortic flow is directed to the umbilical arteries, the aorta is a more accurate reflection of how the fetus is adapting to life *in utero*. This illustration shows aorta waveforms at 24 (a), 32(b), and 36(c) weeks.

not recommended for routine clinical use, measurements obtained in this way can provide information about the fetal circulation.[15] The combined output of the fetal heart at 30 weeks is approximately 550 ml/minute.[16] About 400 ml/minute passes through the thoracic aorta,[17] the remainder supplying the head and neck. About 50% of aortic flow is in turn directed immediately back to the placenta via the umbilical arteries representing approximately 40% of the fetal cardiac output. The well-oxygenated venous return from the placenta passes in the umbilical vein. In the liver umbilical venous blood flow is divided, with half the blood passing into the ductus venosus, and the rest draining into the portal system and hepatic veins.

The limitations of volume flow studies have led us to rely on indices derived from the flow velocity waveform that reflect downstream resistance (e.g. pulsatility index, PI; resistance index, RI), or measurement of peak and time averaged velocities. Much of the work using Doppler-derived indices has been to investigate a possible role for Doppler studies of the fetal circulation in the diagnosis and management of the healthy and complicated pregnancy.

The pulsatility index (PI) of FVWs from the umbil-

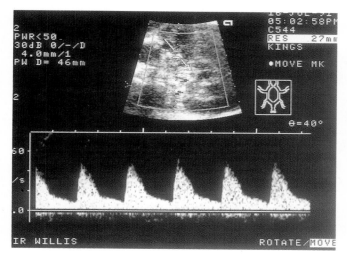

(a)

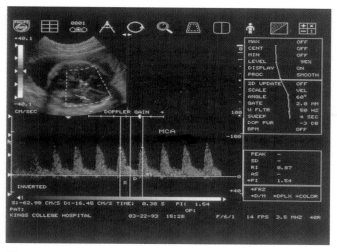

(b)

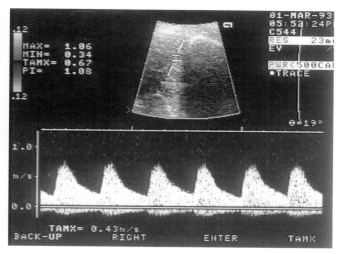

(c)

Fig. 6.22

Unlike the aorta, end diastolic frequencies in the middle cerebral artery continue to increase in the second half of pregnancy, as these images obtained at 24(a), 32(b), and 38(c) weeks illustrate. The fall in middle cerebral resistance is thought to reflect changes in the partial pressure of fetal blood gases through pregnancy. The total amount of fetal haemoglobin rises steadily in the second half of pregnancy, but the partial pressure falls, stimulating the carotid chemoreceptors to increase cerebral flow by reducing cerebral resistance. This effect is exaggerated in the presence of hypoxia. Abnormally low resistance in the middle cerebral arteries is a strong marker for the presence of hypoxia.

ical artery gradually decreases with gestation, and positive EDF is usually present by 16 weeks' gestation (Fig. 6.19). This decrease in resistance is primarily secondary to the increase in the number of tertiary stem villi, and in addition fetal cardiac output. Because the umbilical arteries are arranged in a helical pattern in the cord, a reliable estimate of velocity is not possible. The FVWs may be assessed quantitatively, by the determination of various impedance indices, or qualitatively, by noting the absence or presence of end-diastolic frequencies (EDF), or reverse EDF (Fig. 6.20).

Where it is possible to ascertain the angle of insonation, time averaged velocity (TAV) and peak velocity (Vmax) can be quantified in addition to indices of resistance. For instance, in the aorta the PI remains relatively constant throughout pregnancy (Fig. 6.21), whereas the TAV in the fetal descending thoracic aorta increases with gestation, reaching a plateau in the third trimester.

TAV in vessels that supply the fetal brain, in particular the common carotid and middle cerebral artery (MCA), also increase with gestation (Fig. 6.22). This probably reflects a progressive increase in cardiac output to fulfil the demands of the growing fetus, as TAV and vessel diameter are the parameters used to determine volume flow. The PI, reflecting downstream resistance, while remaining relatively constant in the aorta, steadily falls in the common carotid and MCA. These findings suggest that in the latter part of pregnancy a proportionally greater fraction of the cardiac output is directed to the fetal brain, presumably to compensate for the progressive fall in the partial pressure of fetal blood (pO_2) and to increase the partial pressure (pCO_2). The normal ranges for the umbilical arteries, the middle cerebral arteries and the aorta are presented in the Appendix.

Summary

It has long been recognized that a small or growth-retarded fetus has much greater short-term morbidity and mortality compared with its appropriately grown counterpart. More recently the long-term sequelae of this condition are being recognized, illuminating the importance of the prevention and prediction of pregnancies with fetal growth problems.[18] At present the antenatal assessment of the at risk fetus consists of an estimation of fetal size, amniotic fluid volume and fetal heart rate testing. Identifying smallness or a reduction in growth velocity remains one of our best screening tests of fetal well being. Within a group of small-for-gestational-age (SGA) fetuses there is a higher concentration of complicated pregnancies, but not all fetuses that are SGA are necessarily unwell or abnormal. Fetal heart rate testing is still the primary step in elucidating the nature of the smallness discovered, and if the FHR trace is abnormal it usually confirms that the fetus is in jeopardy. However, in clinical practice, the FHR trace is usually only abnormal or ominous when the fetus is in a terminal state, and there are other signs of compromise. Delaying delivery until the fetus is this unwell may affect subsequent neonatal outcome.[19] The majority of small fetuses will initially have a normal fetal heart rate pattern, regardless of whether the fetus is constitutionally small or sick. This creates difficulties in deciding the frequency and intensity of fetal monitoring that is required for an individual fetus, and generally leads to increased surveillance for all the pregnancies, lest the truly sick fetus be missed.

Doppler studies of the umbilical arteries have been the first step in learning more about the true nature of fetal smallness, and an abnormal umbilical artery PI helps isolate the small sick fetus from the small healthy fetus. But the UA PI primarily informs us about placental resistance, and a fetus can survive with an abnormal UA PI, in relatively good condition, for a variable length of time. Conversely, the umbilical artery waveform can be normal in the presence of fetal arterial redistribution, especially at term. So although a raised UA PI, or the finding of absent or reversed diastolic flow is a big advance compared with relying on the FHR pattern, it will not identify the optimum time for delivering such an at-risk fetus.

Doppler studies of the fetal circulation allow us to see how the fetus is coping with its environment *in utero*. By identifying a pattern of blood flow distribution that suggests hypoxia, changes in the fetal circulation can be monitored. The Chapter 'The fetal haemodynamic response to hypoxia' describes the changes seen in the fetal circulation of the small, sick fetus.

REFERENCES

1 Peeters LLH, Sheldon RE, Jones MD, Makowski EL, Meschia G. (1979) Blood flow to fetal organs as a function of arterial oxygen content. *Am J Obstet Gynecol* **135**: 637–46.

2 Campbell S, Dewhurst CJ. (1971) Diagnosis of the small-for-dates fetus by serial ultrasonic cephalometry. *Lancet* **ii**: 1002–4.

3 Vyas S, Nicolaides KH, Bower S, Campbell S. (1990) Middle cerebral artery flow velocity waveforms in fetal hypoxaemia. *Br J Obstet Gynaecol* **97**: 797–803.

4 Stuart B, Drumm J. Fitzgerald DE, Duignan NM. (1980) Fetal blood velocity waveforms in normal pregnancy. *Br J Obstet Gynaecol* **87**: 780–5.

5 Trudinger BJ, Cook CM et al. (1991) Fetal umbilical artery velocity waveforms and subsequent neonatal outcome. *Br J Obstet Gynaecol* **98**: 378–84.

6 Ruissen CJ, Drongelen HJ, Jager W and Hoeks APG. (1990) Characteristics of the umbilical artery velocity waveform as function of measurement site. *Gynecol Obstet Invest* **30**: 212–16.

7 Bilardo CM, Campbell S, Nicolaides KH. (1988) Mean blood velocities and flow impedance in the fetal descending thoracic aorta and common carotid artery in normal pregnancy. *Early Hum Dev* **18**: 213–18.

8 Meerman RJ, Van Bel F, Van Zwieten PHT et al. (1990) Fetal and neonatal cerebral blood flow velocity in the normal fetus and neonate: a longitudinal Doppler study. *Early Hum Dev* **24**: 209–17.

9 Arduini D, Rizzo G. (1990) Normal values of Pulsatility Index from fetal vessels: a cross sectional study on 1556 healthy fetuses. *J Perinat Med* **18**: 165–71.

10 Van den Wijngaard JAGW, Groenenberg IAL, Wladimiroff JW, Hop WCJ. (1989) Cerebral Doppler ultrasound in the human fetus. *Br J Obstet Gynaecol* **96**: 845–49.

11 Vyas S, Campbell S, Bower S, Nicolaides KH. (1990) Maternal abdominal pressure alters fetal cerebral blood flow. *Br J Obstet Gynaecol* **97**: 740–2.

12 Vyas S, Nicolaides KH, Campbell S. (1989) Renal artery flow velocity waveforms in normal and hypoxemic fetuses. *Am J Obstet Gynecol* **161**: 168–72.

13 Eik-Nes SH, Brubakk AO, Ulstein MK. (1980) Measurement of human fetal blood flow. *Br Med J* **280**: 283–4.

14 Griffin D, Cohen-Overbeek T, Campbell S. (1983) Fetal and uteroplacental blood flow. In: Campbell S (ed.) *Clinics in Obstetrics and Gynaecology* **10**, No. 3: 565–602.

15 Gill RW. Measurement of blood flow by ultrasound. (1985) Accuracy and sources of error. *Ultrasound Med Biol* **11**: 625–31.

16 Griffin DR, Teague MJ et al. (1985) A combined ultrasonic linear array scanner and pulsed Doppler velocimeter for the estimation of blood flow in the fetus and maternal abdomen. *Ultrasound Med Biol* **11**: 37–41.

17 Reed KL, Anderson CF, Shenker L. (1987) Fetal pulmonary artery and aorta: Two-dimensional Doppler echocardiography. *Obstet Gynaecol* **69**:

175–9.

18 Barker DJP. (1992) Fetal growth and adult disease. *Br J Obstet Gynaecol* **99**: 275–6.

19 Soothill PW, Ajayi RA, Campbell S *et al.* (1992) Relationship between fetal acidaemia at cordocentesis and subsequent neurodevelopment. *Ultrasound Obstet Gynecol* **2**: 80–3.

CHAPTER 7

The fetal venous circulation

Kurt Hecher

INTRODUCTION

The first report on measurement of blood flow in the intra-abdominal part of the umbilical vein in human fetuses was published in 1980,[1] shortly after the first description of the use of Doppler ultrasound to obtain signals from the umbilical cord in 1977.[2] This technique was then used to assess umbilical vein volume flow in fetuses affected by rhesus isoimmunization.[3] Although there was a rapid development in the investigation of the fetal arterial circulation (descending aorta, cerebral circulation, renal artery) and the fetal heart by Doppler ultrasound, it was not until this decade that the first reports on other venous fetal vessels (inferior vena cava, ductus venosus) were published. This may be because (i) that it is more difficult to identify these vessels correctly, and (ii) the more complicated waveform of venous blood flow, reflects different pressure–flow relationships throughout the cardiac cycle. This chapter will describe the anatomy and physiology of fetal venous blood flow and the typical blood velocity waveforms that can be recorded from these vessels with blood pulsed Doppler ultrasound will be explained.

ANATOMY

The fetal liver and its venous vasculature is the principal organ determining blood flow to the fetal heart and its distribution between the right and left side of the heart. Ultrasonographic studies have examined the anatomy of these vessels[4, 5] and showed good correlation with findings in fetal postmortems.[6]

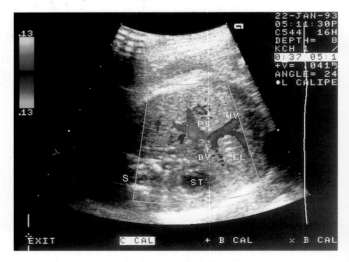

Fig. 7.1
Transverse section through the abdomen. UV = umbilical vein; DV = ductus venosus; PS = portal sinus; LL = left lobe of the liver; ST = stomach. The spine (S) is on the left.

The intra-abdominal part of the umbilical vein (UV) ascends relatively steeply from the cord insertion in the inferior part of the falciform ligament. Then the vessel continues in a more horizontal and posterior direction and turns to the right to the confluence with the transverse left portal vein (also called portal or umbilical sinus), which joins the right portal vein with its division into anterior and posterior branches (Fig. 7.1). Before it becomes the left portal vein, branches of the UV supply the left lobe of the liver (Fig. 7.2) and then the ductus venosus (DV) originates and courses posteriorly and cephalically with increasing steepness in the original direction of the UV (Fig. 7.3). The diameter of the DV is significantly smaller than that of the UV,

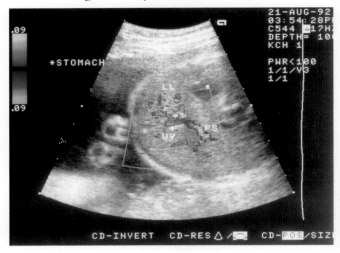

Fig. 7.2
Transverse section through the abdomen. The red signal towards the left lobe (LL) is the supporting branch of the umbilical vein (UV), before it turns right to the portal sinus (PS). The spine is on the right.

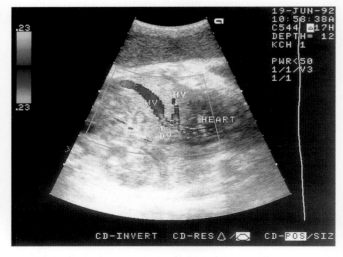

Fig. 7.3
Saggital view of the UV, and the middle hepatic vein (HV)

(approximately one-third).

Other authors identify the posteriorly coursing cephalic part of the UV as the umbilical portion of the left portal vein and criticize that the ultrasound literature commonly mislabels this portion as the UV.[5] Although this may be correct in a strictly anatomical sense, it seems to be more practical to use the term UV as far as the origin of the DV, where the vessel courses abruptly to the right.

The DV enters the inferior vena cava (IVC) before the IVC enters into the right atrium. At the same level the hepatic veins reach the IVC and therefore a sub-diaphragmatic venous vestibulum is formed which has recently been described (Fig. 7.4).[7] It contains the orifices of the hepatic veins and the ductus venosus and forms the most proximal part of the IVC immediately before it enters the right atrium in a slightly anterior direction (Fig. 7.5).

PHYSIOLOGY

The DV plays a central role in the fetal circulation. Well oxygenated blood coming from the placenta flows via this shunt between the UV and the IVC directly towards the heart. There is a considerable variation in the proportion of umbilical venous blood flowing through the DV, but on average approximately 53% of UV blood flow enters the DV and accounts for more than 98% of its blood flow, because portal blood flow is directed almost exclusively to the right lobe of the liver.[8] The oxygen saturation of UV blood and, therefore, of DV blood is about 80–85%, whereas it is only 30–35% in distal IVC blood.

Animal studies have shown that there is streamlining of blood flow within the thoracic IVC.[9] Blood from the DV flows in the dorsal and left part, whereas blood from the lower body flows in the ventral and right part of the IVC. Injections of microspheres labelled with radionuclides demonstrate that these two streams of blood do not mix in the IVC. Blood from the ventral and right stream enters the right atrium and passes through the tricuspid valve into the right ventricle and from there through the main pulmonary artery and the ductus arteriosus to the descending aorta. The dorsal and left stream of IVC blood flow is directed towards

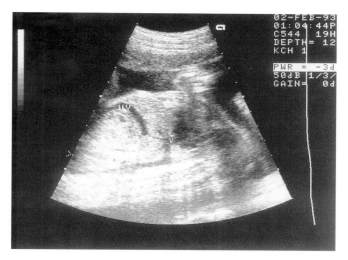

Fig. 7.4
Saggital view of the fetal trunk. The DV enters the venous vestibulum (V) immediately before the right atrium. So do the hepatic veins and the inferior vena cava. The spine is posterior.

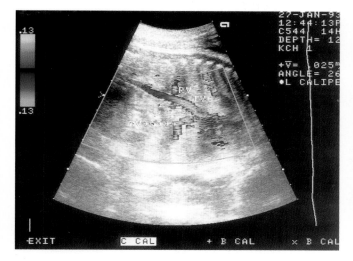

Fig. 7.5
Longitudinal view of the inferior vena cava (IVC) and the ductus venosus (DV) entering it immediately before the right atrium. RV = renal vein. The spine is anterior.

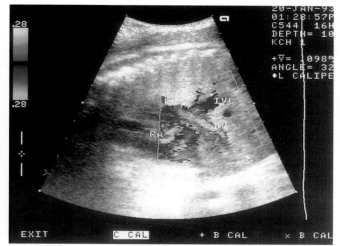

Fig. 7.6
The preferential streaming of blood is shown by the different colour of blood flow from the DV and the distal IVC. The spine is anterior. DV blood flow is coded red and, therefore, directed towards the foramen ovale and the left atrium (LA). IVC blood flow is coded blue. RA = right atrium.

the foramen ovale and therefore delivers well oxygenated blood directly to the left heart and from there via the ascending aorta to the upper part of the body. The preferential streaming of IVC and DV blood in the fetal heart is shown in Figure 7.6.

Blood in the left hepatic veins of the lamb has an oxygen saturation of about 70–75% whereas the saturation of blood in the right hepatic veins is only 50–55%. This is the consequence of well oxygenated blood from the UV supplying the left lobe and a mixture of UV blood and portal vein blood (oxygen saturation about 30%) supplying the right lobe. The right HV blood follows the stream of distal IVC blood flow, whereas left HV blood follows the path of the DV stream[10, 11] (see Fig. 7.15).

As a consequence of this preferential blood streaming, a significantly greater proportion of blood from the DV, rather than IVC blood returning from the lower body and abdominal viscera, supplies the fetal brain and heart. DV blood flow constituted approximately 40% of the total brain and heart perfusion in fetal lambs.[9]

Mechanical factors, such as pressure and resistance differences across the liver, seem to play a major role in the regulation of blood flow through the DV and, therefore, of the proportion of UV blood flow allowed to bypass the liver microcirculation.[12] In fetal lambs it has been shown that a reduction in total umbilical blood flow resulted in an increased proportion of UV blood flow being shunted through the DV, and a decreased proportion to the liver.[13] It was concluded, therefore, that with a reduction in UV pressure, there must have been a relatively greater resistance to blood

flow through the liver than through the DV. This supports the theory that the DV functions passively to maintain an adequate venous return to the fetal heart when UV flow and pressure fluctuate.

On the other hand there also seems to be an active regulation of blood flow through the DV. At the origin of the DV from the UV there is a thickening of the muscular wall which has been described as the sphincter of the DV.[14] Other authors[15] found nerve fibres from the coeliac plexus, the phrenic nerves and the vagal trunks innervating this sphincter in human embryos. Thus sympathetic and parasympathetic innervation also appears to play a role in the regulation of blood flow through the DV.

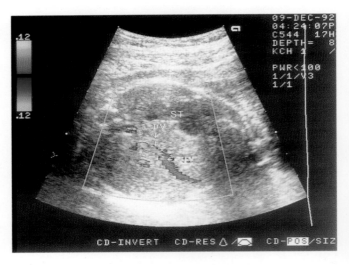

Fig. 7.8
Oblique transverse section through the abdomen showing the UV and DV. The spine is on the left. ST = stomach.

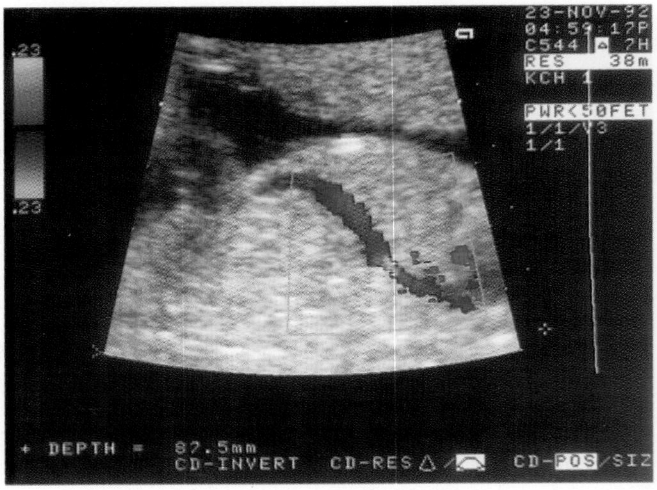

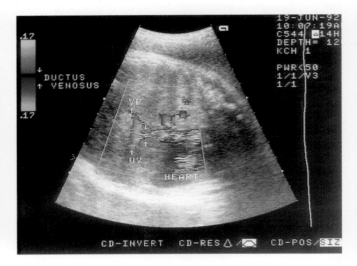

Fig. 7.7
Longitudinal view of the UV and the DV. Note the change from blue to orange and red (aliasing effect) at the origin of the DV. This indicates high velocities.

Fig. 7.9
The origin of the DV is shown at the point where the UV turns towards the venae portae (VP)

Visualization of fetal venous blood flow and its typical Doppler waveforms

The DV can be found with ultrasound either in a mid-sagittal longitudinal section of the fetal trunk (Fig. 7.7), or in an oblique transverse section through the upper abdomen (Figs 7.8 and 7.9). It joins the IVC next to the left HV. Colour Doppler reveals high velocities compared to the UV and sometimes an aliasing effect occurs (Fig. 7.7). This is due to the narrow lumen of the DV (the inner width of the narrowest portion never exceeded 2 mm in a recent ultrasonographic study).[16]

The best ultrasound plane to depict the IVC is a longitudinal or coronal one, where it runs anterior, to the right of and nearly parallel with the descending aorta (Figs 7.5 and 7.10d). The hepatic veins can be visualized either in a transverse section through the upper abdomen, which is slightly less oblique but more cephalic than the plane for the DV (Figs 7.10–7.12), or in a sagittal–coronal section through the respective lobe of the liver (see Fig. 7.3).

Colour Doppler studies in human fetuses confirm the results of animal studies showing preferential blood streaming of DV blood towards the foramen ovale (Fig. 7.13) and blood from the lower IVC and the right HV towards the tricuspid valve (Fig. 7.14). In a recent ultrasonographic study it was shown that the crista dividens, which forms the upper edge of the foramen ovale,

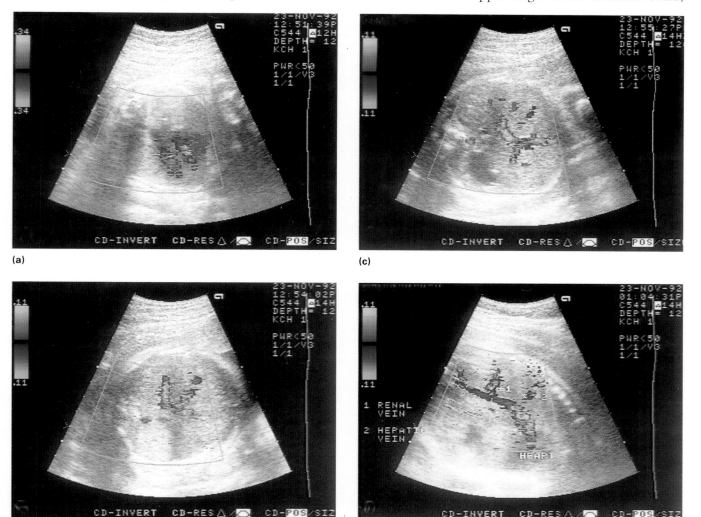

Fig. 7.10
Transverse sections from cranial to caudal (a-c). The spine is on the left side. (a) Fetal heart, both atrioventricular inflow tracts. (b) Hepatic veins. (c) Umbilical vein and portal sinus. The DV can be visualized in an oblique section at its origin only (black arrow). (d) Longitudinal view of the IVC with renal and hepatic vein.

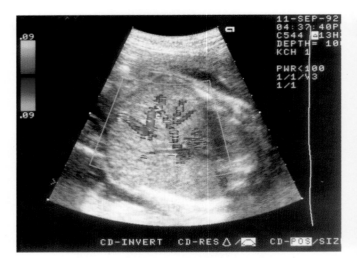

Fig. 7.11
Oblique section; the spine is on the right side. This section is
more oblique than plane (b) and (c) in Fig.7.10 and therefore
shows a combination of both of them with the UV and the
hepatic veins.

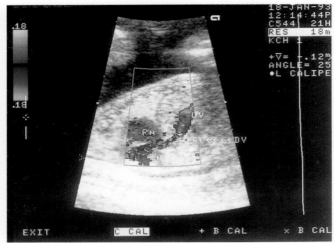

Fig. 7.13
Longitudinal section of the trunk; the spine is posterior. Blood
flow from the DV (blue) is clearly directed downwards through
the foramen ovale towards the left atrium (LA).

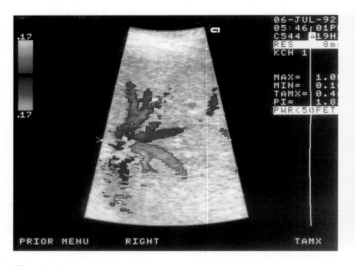

Fig. 7.12
The confluence of the hepatic veins, corresponding to plane (b)
in Fig 7.10

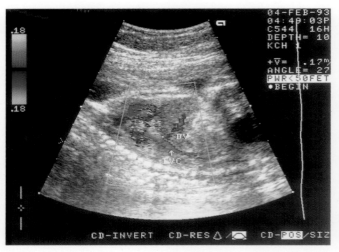

Fig. 7.14
Same section as in Fig 7.13. Blood flow from the distal IVC (red)
is clearly directed towards the anterior thoracic wall and
therefore to the tricuspid valve and the right ventricle.

separates these two pathways and the authors speculate
that blood delivered to the left atrium even circum-
vents the right atrium.[17]

The typical waveforms for blood flow in the DV and
the IVC/HV consist of three phases and their relationship to the cardiac cycle is shown in Figure 7.15. The
highest pressure gradient between the venous vessels
and the right atrium occurs during ventricular systole,
which results in the highest blood flow velocities
(towards the fetal heart) during that part of the cardiac
cycle. Early diastole is associated with a second peak
and the nadir of flow velocities coincides with late
diastole (atrial contraction). There is forward flow in

the DV throughout the whole heart cycle (Figs 7.16
and 7.17). In the IVC there can be forward flow during
atrial contraction (Fig. 7.18) or it can cause absence or
reversal of blood flow (Fig. 7.19), which is almost
always the case in HVs (Fig. 7.20). The percentage of
reverse flow in the IVC decreases with advancing
gestational age.[18] Waveforms of the DV with very little
or even no pulsatility seem to be normal variants and
might be caused by different sphincter activity. They
were found in 3% of measurements in a longitudinal
study of normal pregnancies.[19]

Blood flow velocities in the DV increase with gestational age.[16, 20] The high velocities probably support the

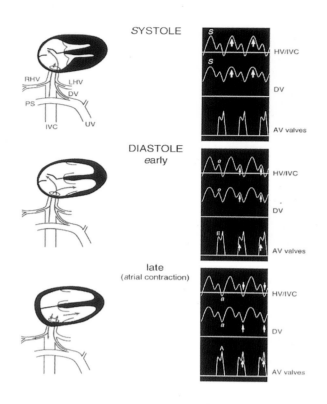

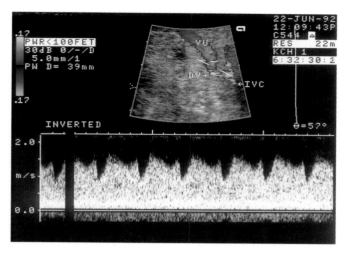

Fig. 7.17
The sample volume is positioned over both the UV and the origin of the DV. Note the abrupt change from non-pulsatile low velocity flow in the UV to pulsative high velocity flow in the DV.

Fig. 7.15
The diagram shows the preferential blood flow of venous return to the fetal heart and the haemodynamics corresponding to systole and diastole. The relevant parts of the venous waveforms and the atrioventricular (AV) inflow are marked with arrows. UV = umbilical vein; DV = ductus venosus; PS = portal sinus; IVC = inferior vena cava; RHV = right hepatic vein; LHV = left hepatic vein.

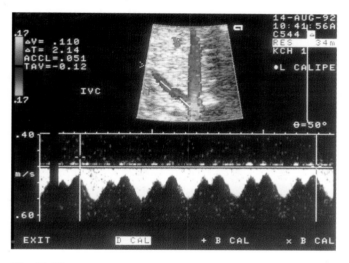

Fig. 7.18
Normal waveform of the IVC with forward flow throughout the heart cycle later in gestation

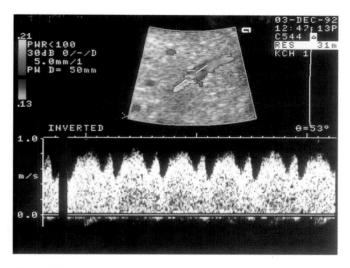

Fig. 7.16
Normal waveform of the ductus venosus. Note the aliasing effect in the colour image.

preferential direction of blood towards the foramen ovale and avoid mixing with blood with a lower oxygen saturation. The mean peak velocities increase from 65 cm/s at 18 weeks to 75 cm/s at term.[16] When measuring DV velocities it is important to standardize the site of sampling. The highest velocities are measured at the inlet of the DV.[19] The nearer to the heart the sampling site is, the higher is the probability of overlap with other venous signals. Therefore, the waveforms should be recorded as near as possible to the UV.

Blood velocity waveforms from the IVC and the HV should be obtained more distal to the venous confluence and right atrium, in order to assess changes in individual venous vessels rather than in the venous

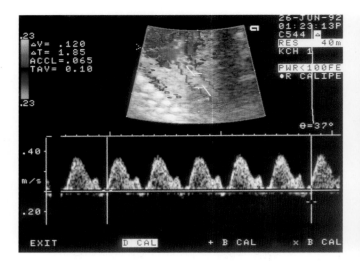

Fig. 7.19
IVC blood flow with a very small percentage of reversed flow with atrial contraction

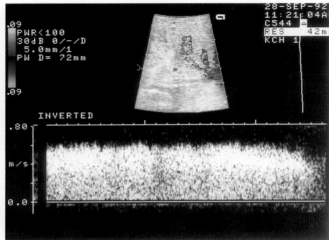

Fig. 7.21
DV blood flow without pulsatility, which seems to be a normal variant

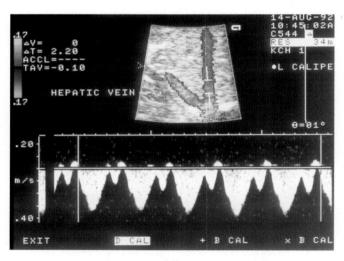

Fig. 7.20
Normal waveform of the HV

vestibulum, which may cause a relatively big variation in velocities with small changes in the scanning plane (Fig. 7.21).[7,18] Fetal breathing movements cause massive changes in venous blood flow velocities and variation in the waveforms during these periods should therefore be avoided for Doppler assessment (Fig. 7.22).

The influence of hypoxia and blood flow redistribution on the venous circulation and the changes of venous Doppler waveforms with fetal compromise will be discussed in Chapter 8.

REFERENCES

1 Eik-Nes SH, Brubakk AO, Ulstein MK. (1980) Measurement of human fetal blood flow. *Br Med J* **280**: 283–4.

2 Fitzgerald DE, Drumm JE. (1977) Non-invasive measurement of human fetal circulation using ultrasound: a new method. *Br Med J* **275**: 1450–1.

3 Kirkinen P, Jouppila P. (1983) Umbilical vein blood flow in rhesus-isoimmunization. *Br J Obstet Gynaecol* **90**: 640–3.

4 Morin R, Winsberg F. (1978) Ultrasonic and radiographic study of the vessels of the fetal liver. *J Clin Ult* **6**: 409–11.

5 Chinn DH, Filly RA, Callen PW. (1982) Ultrasonic evaluation of fetal umbilical and hepatic vascular anatomy. *Radiology* **144**: 153–7.

6 Staudach A. (1987). *Sectional Fetal Anatomy in Ultrasound*. Springer-Verlag, Berlin.

7 Huisman TWA, Gittenberger-de Groot AC, Wladimiroff JW. (1992) Recognition of a fetal subdiaphragmatic venous vestibulum essential for fetal venous Doppler assessment. *Pediat Res* **32**: 338–41.

8 Edelstone DI, Rudolph AM, Heymann MA. (1978) Liver and ductus venosus blood flows in fetal lambs in utero. *Circulat Res* **42**: 426–33.

9 Edelstone DI, Rudolph AM. (1979) Preferential streaming of ductus venosus blood to the brain and heart in fetal lambs. *Am J Physiol* **237**: H724–9.

10 Rudolph AM. (1983) Hepatic and ductus venosus blood flows during fetal life. *Hepatology* **3**: 254–8.

11 Rudolph AM. (1985) Distribution and regulation of blood flow in the fetal and neonatal lamb. *Circulat Res* **57**: 811–21.

12 Edelstone DI. (1980) Regulation of blood flow through the ductus venosus. *J Devel Physiol* **2**: 219–38.

13 Edelstone DI, Rudolph AM, Heymann MA. (1980)

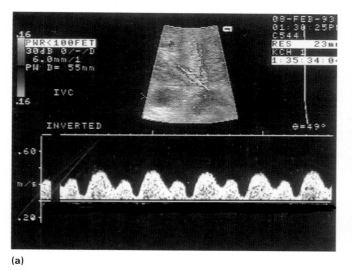

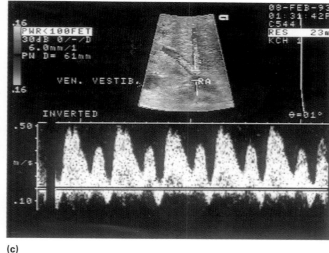

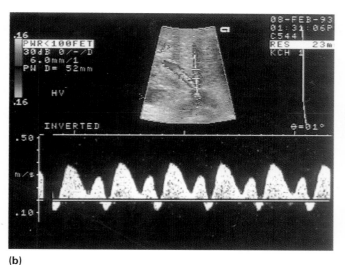

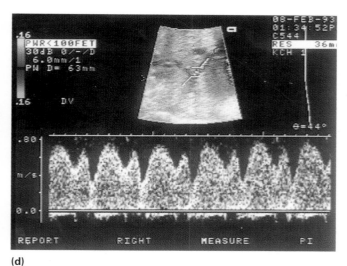

Fig. 7.22
The influence of different sampling sites on the blood flow waveforms. (a) IVC; (b) HV; (d) DV. In (c) the sample volume is positioned in the venous vestibulum before the right atrium. The waveform seems to reflect a combination of the various velocities in (a), (b) and (d), and is not typical for any of the individual vessels.

Effects of hypoxemia and decreasing umbilical flow on liver and ductus venosus blood flows in fetal lambs. *Am J Physiol* **238**: H656–63.

14 Barron DH. (1942) The 'sphincter' of the ductus venosus. *J Anatomy* **82**: 398.

15 Pearson AA, Sauter RW. (1971) Observations on the phrenic nerves and the ductus venosus in human embryos and fetuses. *Am J Obstet Gynecol* **110**: 560–5.

16 Kiserud T, Eik-Nes SH, Blaas HGK, Hellevik LR. (1991) Ultrasonographic velocimetry of the fetal ductus venosus. *Lancet* **338**: 1412–14.

17 Kiserud T, Eik-Nes SH, Blaas HG, Hellevik LR. (1992) Foramen ovale: an ultrasonographic study of its relation to the inferior vena cava, ductus venosus and hepatic veins. *Ultrasound Obstet Gynecol* **2**: 389–96.

18 Huisman TWA, Stewart PA, Wladimiroff JW. (1991) Flow velocity waveforms in the fetal inferior vena cava during the second half of normal pregnancy. *Ult Med Biol* **17**: 679–82.

19 Kiserud T, Eik-Nes SH, Hellevik LR, Blaas HG. (1992) Ductus venosus – a longitudinal Doppler velocimetric study of the human fetus. *J Matern Fet Invest* **2**: 5–11.

20 Huisman TWA, Stewart PA, Wladimiroff JW. (1992) Ductus venosus blood flow velocity waveforms in the human fetus – a Doppler study. *Ult Med Biol* **18**: 33–7.

CHAPTER 8

The fetal haemodynamic response to hypoxia

Kevin Harrington, Kurt Hecher and Stuart Campbell

INTRODUCTION

Physiological changes in the fetal circulation have already been described in Chapters 6 and 7. This chapter will map the changes that can be observed using current Doppler technology in both the arterial and venous compartments of the fetal and umbilical circulation. The introduction of colour Doppler imaging (CDI)/duplex systems has enabled the more detailed examination of the fetal circulation, thereby allowing a greater knowledge of the physiological and pathophysiological changes in the fetus during pregnancy.

Being small at birth is associated with greater short and long term[1] morbidity and mortality.[1] Doppler ultrasound of the fetal circulation allows us to investigate the fetal response to adverse conditions *in utero*. This

![Sequential changes in tests of fetal well being in uteroplacental failure]

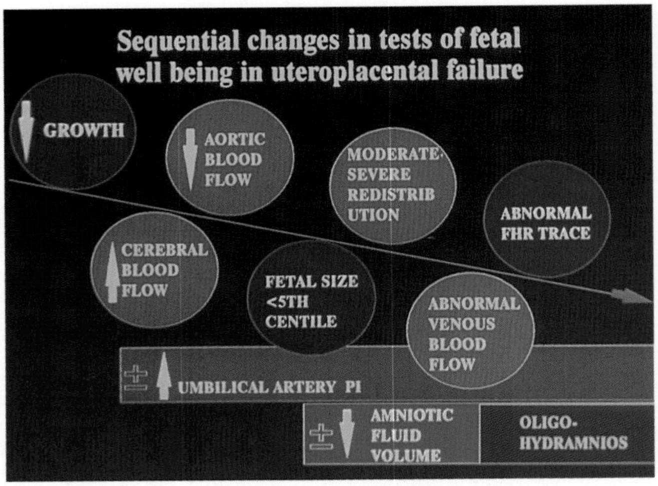

Fig. 8.1
A diagrammatic representation of the typical sequence of changes in investigations of the fetus compromized by chronic uteroplacental insufficiency. When a fetus is faced with a reduced supply of nutrients, it can maintain basal metabolism by reducing growth velocity. If there is a reduced supply of oxygen, increased cerebral flow can be achieved by reducing cerebral vascular resistance. Constriction of the central circulation (aorta) and ultimately cardiovascular collapse (venous and fetal heart rate changes) will follow if there is no intervention.

information can only help in defining the small baby that is sick[2] and may also be useful in determining when it is better to have the fetus delivered, rather than remain *in utero*. The primary response observed with fetal Doppler is the 'brain-sparing' effect which has been demonstrated in both animal[3] and human[4] studies. It has been possible to correlate the development of hypoxia and acidosis with changes in fetal haemodynamics that correspond to the brain-sparing effect, whereby the blood supply (and thereby oxygen and nutrients) is preferentially supplied to the fetal heart, adrenal glands and brain, at the expense of the rest of

the body.

The sequence of change in fetal Doppler ultrasound and other tests of well-being are now being appreciated in the at-risk fetus.[5] The typical sequence of change in fetal tests in the compromised fetus is illustrated in Figure 8.1. This chapter proposes to illustrate the Doppler observed changes in the fetal circulation in the compromised fetus. The haemodynamic response of the fetus to anaemia is also described.

THE FETAL ARTERIAL CIRCULATION IN THE SGA FETUS

The response to hypoxaemia and acidaemia

THE UMBILICAL ARTERIAL CIRCULATION

There is a reduction in the number of arterioles in the tertiary stem villi in pregnancies complicated with fetal growth retardation (IUGR).[6] It is probable that high resistance waveforms in the umbilical arteries (UA) reflects this finding, in addition to the problems of infarction and thrombosis seen in the placental bed of such pregnancies (Fig. 8.2).[7] The waveform can be assessed qualitatively by noting the presence or absence of end diastolic frequencies (EDF) (Fig. 8.2) or quantitatively by measuring an index of resistance (Fig. 8.3). Although the use of the UA FVW as a screening test in low risk populations has been shown to be of limited value,[8] high resistance UA FVWs are associated with an increased risk of a fetus being chromosomally abnormal,[9] especially if discovered in combination with

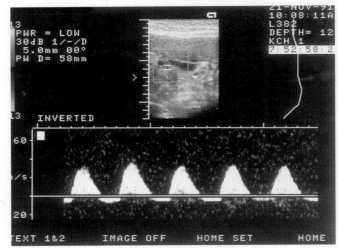

Fig. 8.2
An umbilical artery (UA) waveform, showing reverse end diastolic frequencies (EDF). Whereas absent EDF may exist for a variable length of time before the fetus succumbs, reversed EDF is an ominous sign indicating that the fetus is not likely to survive *in utero* for very long.

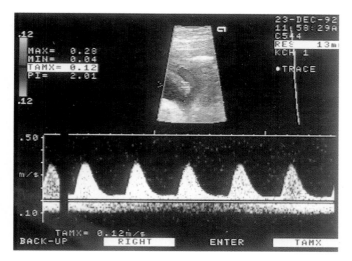

Fig. 8.3
Although there is positive EDF in this UA waveform, it is clearly high resistance for this gestation (34 weeks) and the RI and PI are > 95th centile. This is an abnormal UA FVW that requires further investigation, as it is likely that there is some degree of compromize within the fetus.

structural anomalies.[10] An increase in perinatal morbidity and mortality, irrespective of the fetus being chromosomally abnormal, has also been demonstrated.[11] It is not surprising therefore that an analysis of 207 SGA pregnancies found absent UA EDF in 119 cases and in 87 of these patients (73%) the fetal blood pO_2 was below the 25th centile of the normal range.[12]

Umbilical artery Doppler measurements are now an essential part of determining the aetiology of fetal smallness. Because the UA does not inform us about how the fetus is coping with a compromized supply, it

will not identify all the compromized fetuses in a population and thus it is not the best test to determine the optimum time for delivery. Furthermore, because of the increased risk of chromosomal abnormality in fetuses with absent or reversed UA EDF, it is necessary to consider karyotyping prior to a decision about delivery. If the pregnancy has reached more than 32 weeks' gestation, it would seem reasonable to consider delivery of a fetus with absent UA EDF. Reverse UA EDF is usually a preterminal event and is a stronger indication for delivery, unless the fetus is not viable.

Although UA Doppler is not the ideal Doppler index to manage a pregnancy, it may be more useful than the conventional management of an SGA fetus (serial fetal heart rate tracing). In a randomized trial umbilical artery Doppler tests were more valuable than fetal heart rate tracing in the management of the SGA fetus,[13] although in practice both tests are employed.

THE AORTA AND COMMON CAROTID ARTERIES

It is the condition of the fetus that really concerns us. It is logical to suppose that fetal Doppler measurements are likely to reflect more accurately how the fetus is adapting to its environment *in utero*. Blood flow in the fetal aorta reflects cardiac output and peripheral resistance within the fetus and placenta.[14] The pattern of aortic flow in healthy and complicated pregnancies has already been reported (Fig. 8.4).[15] The relationship between fetal acid/base status (obtained at cordocentesis) and changes in the fetal circulation have been investigated to help with our understanding of the events that are observed with fetal Doppler ultrasound.

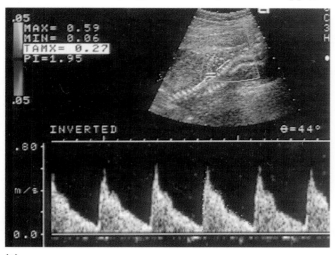

(a)

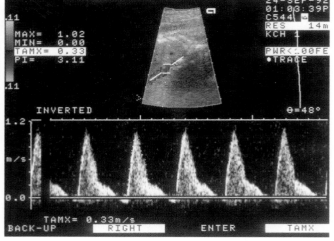

(b)

Fig. 8.4
There is usually positive EDF in the FVW from the thoracic aorta during the second half of pregnancy. (a) With moderate to severe redistribution, there is elevated resistance with eventual loss of EDF, (b). This usually represents significant compromize within the fetal circulation. With restriction of the fetal arterial circulation there is an increase in cardiac afterload.

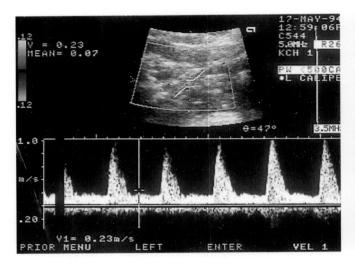

Fig. 8.5

The common carotid artery can be visualized as it leaves the aortic arch and ascends into the neck. Before the introduction of colour Doppler imaging (CDI), it was the most useful vessel for examining changes in the circulation to the fetal head. The middle cerebral artery (MCA) can be visualized quite easily with CDI and has become the preferred vessel for interrogation (see Fig. 8.8).

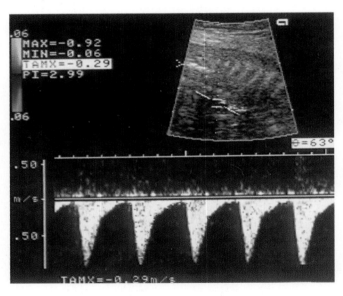

Fig. 8.6

In addition to an increase in resistance in the fetal aorta, there is a reduction in time averaged velocity (TAV), as can be seen in this typical example of a growth-retarded fetus. Compare this with the TAV from the aorta FVW of an anaemic fetus in Fig. 8.22.

The PI and time averaged velocities (TAV) of the fetal aorta and common carotid artery (Fig. 8.6) have been correlated with fetal pH, pCO_2 and pO_2.[3] There were significant correlations between the blood gas result and both the PI and TAV in the individual vessels (Fig. 8.6), but the best correlation was found with the

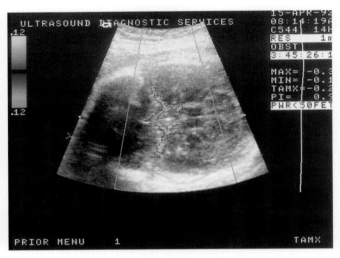

Fig. 8.7

CDI of the circle of Willis. This image can be easily obtained by sliding the transducer down from the plane of the biparietal diameter.

ratio of the common carotid artery and descending thoracic aorta. In this analysis the best predictor of asphyxia (as judged by an asphyxia index calculated from the pH, pCO_2 and pO_2) was the aorta TAV/carotid artery PI index. A normal index was always associated with normal blood gases.

There is a significant relationship between fetal acidaemia and absence of EDF in the aorta.[16] This probably reflects the 'lower limb' or 'hind quarter' reflex seen in animal studies, which indicates significant vasoconstriction of the peripheral circulation. It is thought that this is an endstage mechanism designed to ensure adequate supply of nutrients to the brain in the face of a dramatically diminished supply, when cerebral vasodilatation is not enough to maintain an adequate supply of oxygen and nutrients to the fetal brain. Absent EDF in the aorta is associated with an increase in neonatal complications, most noticeably necrotizing enterocolitis.[17] It is probable that the relationship exists because reduced blood flow results in hypoperfusion of the fetal gut and liver.

THE MIDDLE CEREBRAL ARTERY

The common carotid artery (Fig. 8.6) supplies the tissues of the head and neck in addition to the brain, so investigation of the cerebral circulation may yield more precise information than the carotid arteries about changes in the circulation of the fetal brain. With colour flow imaging it is possible to visualize the cerebral circulation (Fig. 8.7) and identify and obtain measurements from the middle cerebral artery (MCA) (Fig. 8.8). Change in PI and TAV values from that vessel have been correlated with fetal blood gas results in SGA fetuses.[19] The MCA PI was significantly lower

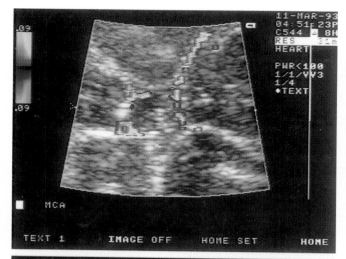

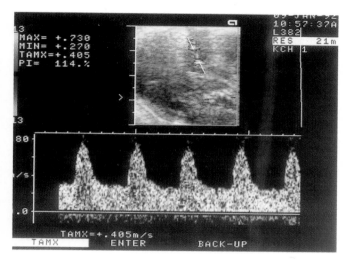

Fig. 8.9
A low resistance FVW from the MCA of a growth retarded, hypoxic fetus at 0 weeks. The first response of the fetus to hypoxia appears to be a reduction in cerebral resistance, which allows an increase in cerenral flow without increasing systemic resistance.

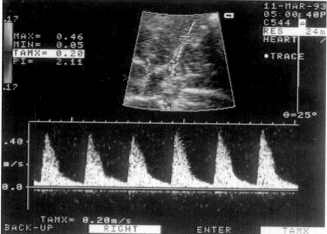

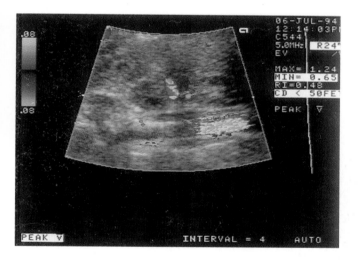

Fig. 8.8
FVW of the MCA in a normally grown fetus in the third trimester. Although there is normally an increase in diastolic frequencies in the third trimester, the findings in redistribution are usually more profound.

Fig. 8.10
CDI of the abdominal aorta and renal arteries. With the transducer in this plane it is usually possible to obtain a satisfactory image of the renal artery FVW.

(Fig. 8.9) and the MCA TAV significantly higher than the reference range in the SGA fetuses. These data provide evidence of vasodilatation in the cerebral vasculature during mild to moderate hypoxia. With severe degrees of hypoxia (2–4 standard deviations below the normal mean for gestation), usually with associated acidosis, the reduction in PI reaches a maximum, which probably represents maximum vessel dilatation.

THE RENAL ARTERY

The renal artery can be examined when obtaining a longitudinal view of the fetus, such that the aortic bifurcation is visible (Fig. 8.10). Doppler indices from the renal artery (RA) have also been measured in SGA fetuses.[20] The renal artery PI in SGA fetuses was significantly higher than the normal mean for gestation

(Fig. 8.11), but a significant relationship between RA PI and pO_2 could not be established. Interestingly in the subgroup of fetuses investigated after 24 weeks' gestation there was a significant association between RA PI and pO_2.

As the primary source of amniotic fluid after 16 weeks' gestation is fetal urine, the relationship between the RA PI and oligohydramnios (vertical diameter of the largest pool of amniotic fluid less than 1 cm) was also investigated. Again there was no significant difference in the mean RA PI between the patients with and

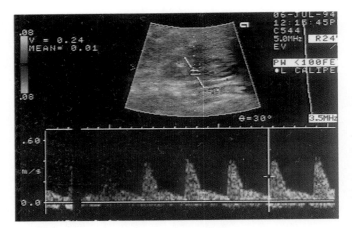

Fig. 8.11
A renal artery waveform from a well grown fetus in the third trimester. The renal artery is a less useful predictor of hypoxia/acidosis because the FVW may be high resistance in the normal pregnancy. It has been used successfully in the management of the anaemic fetus.

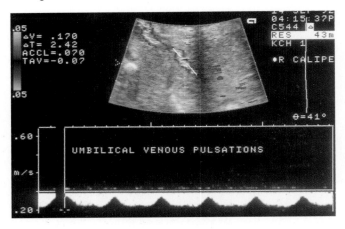

Fig. 8.12
Pulsations in intra-abdominal umbilical vein blood flow. The lowest flow velocity coincides with atrial contraction.

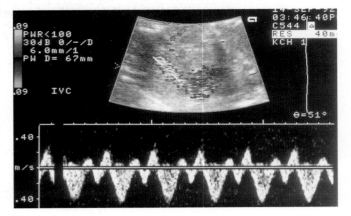

Fig. 8.13
Abnormal blood flow waveform in the inferior vena cava. The reversed flow during atrial contraction exceeds early diastolic forward flow and there is also reversed flow between systolic and early diastolic forward flow.

without oligohydramnios. In SGA pregnancies investigated after 24 weeks' gestation, the renal artery PI was above the 95th centile of the reference range in 15 (94%) of 16 pregnancies in which an ultrasound diagnosis of oligohydramnios was made. However, in the same group, oligohydramnios was present in only 15 (54%) of the 28 pregnancies in which the renal artery PI was above the 95th centile of the reference range. It is probably that an elevated RA PI reflects systemic vascular changes and although oligohydramnios is likely to be in part a consequence of altered fetal renal blood flow, the RA PI does not always reflect this.

THE INFLUENCE OF HYPOXIA ON FETAL VENOUS BLOOD FLOW

Animal experiments suggest that during hypoxia the percentage of umbilical venous blood which bypasses the liver through the ductus venosus (DV) increases, thereby increasing the proportion of umbilical vein (UV) blood contributing to the fetal cardiac output during hypoxaemia. This results in a doubling of UV derived oxygen delivery to the myocardium[21] and a 50% increase in oxygen delivery to the fetal brain. This preference for shunting blood through the DV can also be seen in term primate fetuses.[22] As other authors have not found hypoxaemia capable of altering liver and DV blood flows in the fetal lamb it is not clear what the mechanism for shunting is in growth retarded hypoxic fetuses.[23] Different animal experiments have shown that there is an increase in the amplitude of vena caval pulsations during hypoxaemia and an increased afterload, caused by an increase in peak systolic flow and retrograde flow during atrial contraction.[24] In contrast, reductions in afterload were associated with an increase in peak diastolic forward flow.

The conclusion of these occasionally conflicting animal experiments is that severe hypoxaemia combined with acidosis causes redistribution of UV blood towards the DV at the expense of hepatic blood flow and that fetal systemic vascular resistance has a major influence on venous return and filling patterns of the right heart. Peripheral vasoconstriction, as seen in fetal arterial redistribution, causes an increase in ventricular afterload and thus ventricular end diastolic pressure increases. This results in retrograde blood flow in the IVC with atrial contraction. Pulsations in UV blood flow can occur in the same circumstances.

In the human UV pulsations are a normal finding in the first trimester,[25] but later in pregnancy they are an ominous sign indicating a deterioration in cardiac function (Fig. 8.12). In the viable fetus UV pulsations are associated with severe growth retardation, absent

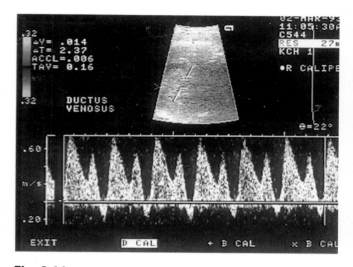

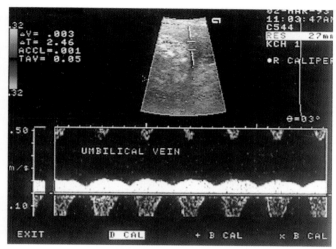

Fig. 8.14
Abnormal ductus venosus blood flow waveform, with reversed flow during atrial contraction. This in turn causes pulsations (which coincide with late diastole) in the umbilical vein. The waveform with a high resistance arterial flow pattern (absent EDF) in the opposite channel was recorded in a free loop of the cord.

end diastolic velocities in the umbilical artery (UA), abnormal fetal heart rates and non-immune hydrops.[26-29] In all these studies abnormal waveforms were also found in the IVC with an increase in the percentage of blood flowing in a reverse direction during atrial contraction (Fig. 8.13). In cases with non-immune hydrops the right ventricular shortening fraction was significantly decreased, thus indicating chronic congestive heart failure. If UV pulsations are seen in addition to absent UA EDF and/or non-immune hydrops the mortality is 64%, with a very high associated morbidity.[27,29]

A decrease in right ventricular fractional shortening in combination with an increase in the ratio of the right to left ventricular end diastolic diameters was also reported in a group of 13 third trimester pregnancies with absence of end diastolic velocities in the fetal descending thoracic aorta.[30] Thus severe intrauterine compromise appears to be associated with right ventricular dysfunction, independent of and often without changes in left ventricular function. As with alterations in the arterial system, these changes precede subsequent abnormalities in the fetal heart trace or cardiotocograph (CTG).

These observations may explain the finding that in SGA fetus with abnormal UA PI values, there is a

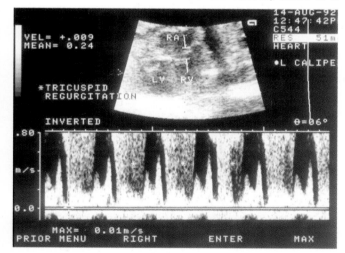

Fig. 8.15
Highly pulsatile waveform of the ductus venosus in a severely growth retarded fetus at 28 weeks. There is a reversal of blood flow with atrial contraction and a decrease in early diastolic forward velocities. Fetal blood gas analysis after cordocentesis revealed severe hypoxaemia and acidaemia.

Fig. 8.16
Tricuspid regurgitation in a recipient twin case of twin to twin transfusion syndrome. The sample volume is placed over the tricuspid valve. The Doppler signals are inverted.
Atrioventricular inflow shows the typical two peaks (E-and A-wave), followed by pansystolic regurgitation. RA = right atrium; RV = right ventricle; LV = left ventricle.

significantly higher ratio between peak systolic and diastolic velocities and a higher percentage of reverse flow with atrial contraction in the IVC, compared to an SGA fetus with normal UA flow.[31] In SGA fetuses with high resistance flow patterns in the UA studied longitudinally, a progressive change in IVC waveforms preceded the onset of late heart rate decelerations. The same group of authors reported that, besides gestational age and the presence of hypertension, pulsatile blood flow in the UV was the dominant factor determining the length of the interval between the first occurrence of absent end diastolic velocities in the UA and the development of late heart rate decelerations and delivery.[32] This was the result of a multivariate analysis including ten different fetal Doppler measurements in a group of 37 fetuses with absent end diastolic velocities in the UA. The incidence of UV pulsations was 43%; the neonatal mortality in this group was 63% compared to 19% in fetuses without pulsations.

Umbilical venous and arterial flow are interdependent and influenced by alterations in placental and ventricular filling.[33] This, and the fact that changes in right ventricular function are transmitted to the UV via the DV, suggests that measuring DV blood flow may be of use in investigating the compromised fetus (Fig. 8.14). Significant changes in ductus venous Doppler waveforms (reversed a wave) develop after fetal arterial redistribution is established and appear to be closely related to abnormal biophysical assessment. Doppler investigation of the fetal venous circulation may play an important role in monitoring the redistributing, growth retarded fetus and, thereby, help to determine the optimal time for delivery.[34]

As already mentioned in Chapter 7 there is forward flow with high velocities in the DV throughout the cardiac cycle. However, the lowest velocities are seen with atrial contraction and with progressing fetal hypoxia they decrease significantly. In cases with severe hypoxaemia and acidaemia, DV velocities with atrial contraction can be reduced to zero or even become negative, indicating a reversal of blood flow (Fig. 8.15). The increased pulsatility is then transmitted beyond the DV, causing pulsatile waveforms in the intra-abdominal part of the UV and even in free loops of the cord. The same phenomenon occurs in cases of twin–twin transfusion syndrome, with the development of right heart failure in the recipient (Fig. 8.16), which in this instance is a consequence of cardiac overload due to hypervolaemia.

THE SEQUENCE OF CHANGES IN THE FETAL CIRCULATION

From the preceding sections it is clear that the fetal circulation undergoes a sequence of change in response to hypoxaemia (see Fig. 8.1). The initial response observed with Doppler ultrasound is cerebral vascular dilatation (Fig. 8.17). This encourages an increased flow of blood with the highest oxygen concentration to the developing fetal brain. If this response is insufficient the systemic arterial resistance (as represented by the aorta) rises, with eventual loss of end diastolic frequencies (Fig. 8.18). These changes will typically be accompanied by abnormal UA flow, but the UA PI can be

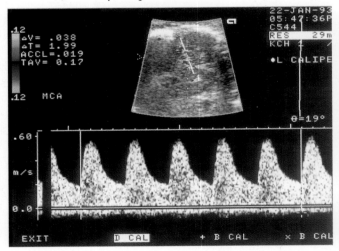

Fig. 8.17
The first step in increasing cerebral flow is a reduction in cerebral vascular resistance. In the SGA fetus this finding suggests that there is some degree of redistribution. If resistance and velocities in the aorta are normal this suggests hypoxia without acidaemia.

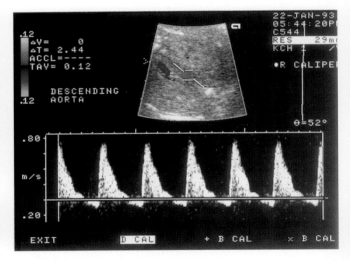

Fig. 8.18
If cerebral vascular dilatation is not sufficient to maintain adequate myocardial and cerebral oxygenation, systemic and peripheral vasoconstriction occurs. Qualitatively this is represented by the finding of absent EDF in the thoracic aorta.

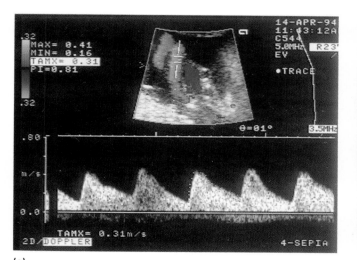

(a)

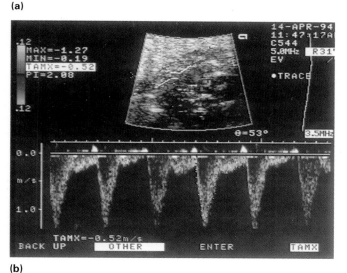

(b)

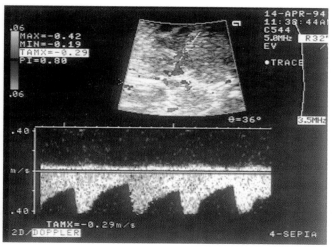

(c)

Fig. 8.19

In the later stages of pregnancy the UA PI may be normal in the presence of redistribution. In this growth retarded fetus at 35 weeks the UA PI is within the normal range (a), but the aorta PI is elevated (b) (and the MCA PI low (c)). It is important to investigate the fetal circulation when assessing the SGA fetus.

normal in the presence of arterial redistribution (Fig. 8.19). Venous Doppler studies become abnormal at a later stage. Figure 8.20 illustrates this sequence by showing arterial redistribution with normal venous flow patterns. The increased afterload, especially on the right side of the heart, is ultimately manifest in the changes seen in the IVC, DV and hepatic veins (Fig. 8.21). It is at this stage that the fetus has become severely compromised and an abnormal fetal heart rate pattern, indicating cerebrovascular collapse, usually follows within days.

Fetal anaemia

Fetal anaemia is typically a consequence of rhesus or other blood group incompatibility. Anaemia results in a decrease in the volume of oxygen carried per ml of blood, but does not affect the partial pressures of oxygen and carbon dioxide. The fetus therefore increases cardiac output without redistributing blood flow pref-

erentially to the brain. Doppler studies have been able to demonstrate a relationship between flow velocities and fetal haematrocrit.[35] Velocities in the fetal aorta are also elevated (Fig. 8.22) and this finding can help in the management of the anaemic fetus, identifying when it is appropriate to perform cordocentesis for the purpose of checking the haemoglobin level and performing an intrauterine blood transfusion.[36] The effects of intrauterine transfusion can also be assessed with Doppler ultrasound in the fetal heart[37] and peripheral circulation.[38] These studies confirm the effect of transfusion on relieving the hyperdynamic state created by the anaemia.

SUMMARY

Doppler studies of the fetal circulation therefore allow us to determine, with a non-invasive test, the ability of the fetus to cope with the environment *in utero*. The

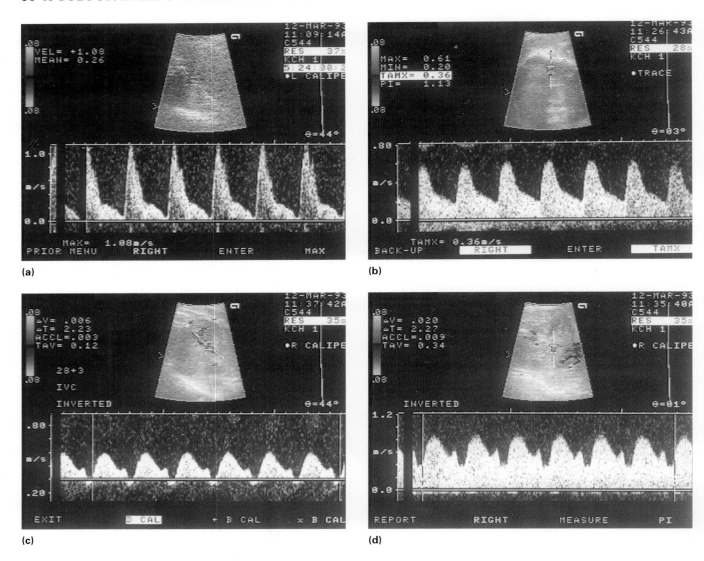

(a)

(b)

(c)

(d)

Fig. 8.20

Top: Fetal arterial blood flow redistribution at 28 weeks. The descending thoracic aorta shows low end diastolic velocities (a), whereas the middle cerebral artery shows a marked increase in end diastolic velocities (b). This indicates that there is moderate to severe arterial redistribution. *Bottom:* Normal venous blood flow patterns from the inferior vena cava (c) and the ductus venosus (d), obtained from the same patient.

first response of a fetus faced with a reduced supply of nutrients from the placenta is to reduce its metabolic needs by slowing growth velocity. This is coupled with an increase in cerebral blood flow, the first Doppler sign that compensation is required. Maximal cerebral flow is reached approximately 2 weeks before the onset of fetal heart rate decelerations, but fetal systemic changes in blood flow redistribution continue until delivery.

The severity of fetal redistribution of blood flow is a guide to the degree of adaptation required of the fetus and there is a good correlation between loss of end diastolic frequencies in the aorta and the development

of acidaemia. Arterial blood flow redistribution in the face of a reduced supply of oxygen and nutrients provides sufficient oxygen supply to the brain and the myocardium. As long as the fetus is able to maintain this compensatory mechanism, preferential myocardial oxygenation delays development of right heart failure, despite an increased afterload. Therefore, fetal Doppler measurements may show arterial redistribution in the presence of normal venous waveforms. The majority of these fetuses have normal, reactive heart rate traces and normal biophysical profiles at this stage.

Progressive changes in the venous circulation signal a failure of the compensatory mechanism and the devel-

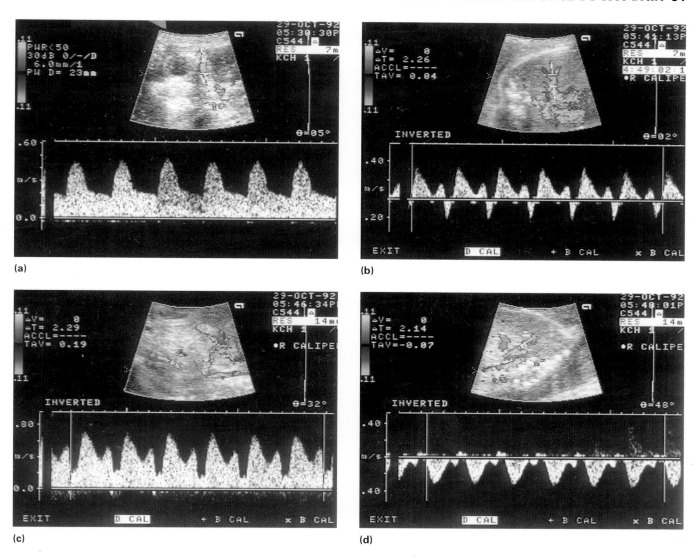

Fig. 8.21
Fetal arterial redistribution at 27 weeks, with a low resistance (increased end diastolic velocities) in the middle cerebral artery (a). The right hepatic vein (b) shows marked reversed flow with atrial contraction. There is also low forward flow during early and late diastole in the ductus venosus (c) and very low forward flow during early diastole in the inferior vena cava (d). The venous changes indicate failure of myocardial function.

opment of right heart failure due to an increased after-load and myocardial hypoxia. An abnormal CTG typically occurs soon afterwards. Serial Doppler studies of the fetal arterial and venous circulation can chronicle the rate and degree of compensation required of the fetus in the face of a reduction in metabolic supply and alert us to the fact that the fetus can no longer cope *in utero*. This information is likely to be of fundamental importance in the assessment of the growth retarded fetus. It has already become an essential part of our investigation of the SGA fetus. However, if fetal Doppler results are to become the primary criteria for delivery, prospective management studies will be required to evaluate the value of this approach.

REFERENCES

1 Harrington K, Campbell S. (1993) Fetal size and growth. *Curr Opin Obstet Gynaecol* **5**: 186-94.
2 Hecher K, Spernol R, Stettner H, Szalay S. (1992) Potential for diagnosing imminent risk to appropriate and small for gestational age fetuses by Doppler sonographic examination of umbilical and cerebral blood flow. *Ult Obstet Gynecol* **2**: 266–71.
3 Bilardo CM, Nicolaides KH, Campbell S. (1990) Doppler measurement of fetal and uteroplacental

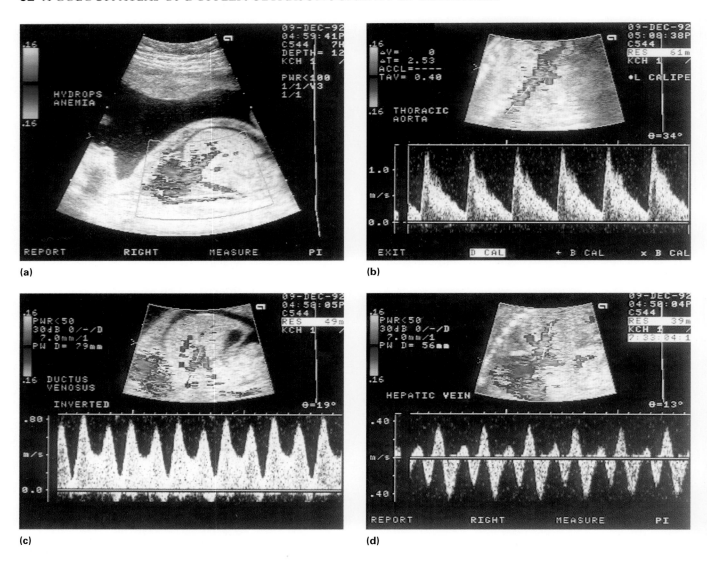

Fig. 8.22
Blood flow studies in a hydropic fetus (a), due to anaemia at 23 weeks. Velocities in the aorta (b) are significantly increased (40 cm/s). The waveforms in the ductus venosus (c) and the hepatic vein (d) show both high velocities and a pulsatile waveform.

circulations: relationship with umbilical venous blood gases measured at cordocentesis. *Am J Obstet Gynecol* **162**: 115–20.

4 Peeters LLH, Sheldon RE, Jones MD, Makowski EL, Meschia G. (1979) Blood flow to fetal organs as a function of arterial oxygen content. *Am J Obstet Gynecol* **135**: 637–46.

5 Arduini D, Rizzo G, Romanini C. (1992) Changes of pulsatility index from fetal vessels preceding the onset of late decelerations in growth-retarded fetuses. *Obstet Gynaecol* **79**: 605–10.

6 Giles WB, Trudinger BJ, Baird PJ. (1985) Fetal umbilical artery flow velocity waveforms and placental resistance: pathological correlation. *Br J Obstet Gynaecol* **92**: 31–8.

7 Trudinger BJ, Cook CM *et al.* (1991) Fetal umbilical artery velocimetry waveforms and subsequent neonatal outcome. *Br J Obstet Gynaecol* **98**: 378–84.

8 Beattie RB, Dornan JC. (1989) Antenatal screening for intrauterine growth retardation with umbilical artery Doppler ultrasonography. *Br Med J* **298**: 631–5.

9 Wenstrom KD, Weiner CP, Williamson RA. (1991) Diverse maternal and fetal pathology associated with absent diastolic flow in the umbilical artery of high risk fetuses. *Obstet Gynaecol* **77**: 374–8.

10 Hecher K, Spernol D, Wimmer-Hebein D, Zierler H, Szalay S. (1992) Doppler sonography of the umbilical artery in fetuses with abnormal ultrasound findings and/or chromosomal abnormal-

ities. *Geburtsh u. Fraeunheilk* **52**: 275–82.

11 Trudinger BJ, Cook CM *et al.* (1991) Fetal umbilical artery velocimetry waveforms and subsequent neonatal outcome. *Br J Obstet Gynaecol* **98**: 378–84.

12 Campbell S, Vyas S, Nicolaides KH. (1991) Doppler investigation of the fetal circulation. *J Perinat Med* **19**: 21–6.

13 Almstrom H, Axelson O, Cnattinghius S *et al.* (1992) Comparison of umbilical artery velocimetry and cardiotocography for surveillance of small for gestational fetuses. *Lancet* **340**: 936–40.

14 Lingman G, Marsal K. (1986) Fetal central blood circulation in the third trimester of normal pregnancy. II Aorta blood velocity waveforms. *Early Hum Devel* **13**: 151–9.

15 Jouppila P, Kirkin P. (1986) Blood velocity waveforms of the fetal aorta in normal and hypertensive pregnancies. *Obstet Gynaecol* **67**: 856–60.

16 Akalin-Sel T, Nicolaides KH, Campbell S. (1992) Understanding the pathophysiology of intrauterine growth retardation: the role of the lower limb reflex in redistribution of blood flow. *Eur J Obstet. Gynecol* **46**: 2–4.

17 Hackett GAS, Campbell S, Gamsu H, Cohen-Overbeek T, Pearce JMF. (1987) Doppler studies in the growth retarded fetus and prediction of neonatal necrotising enterocolitis, haemorrhage and neonatal morbidity. *Br Med J* **294**: 13–16.

18 Van den Wijngaard JAGW, Groenenberg IAL, Wladimiroff JW, Hop WCJ. (1989) Cerebral Doppler ultrasound in the human fetus. *Br J Obstet Gynaecol* **96**: 845–9.

19 Vyas S, Nicolaides KH, Bower S, Campbell S. (1990) Middle cerebral artery flow velocity waveforms in fetal hypoxaemia. *Br J Obstet Gynaecol* **97**: 797–803.

20 Vyas S, Nicolaides KH, Campbell S. (1989) Renal artery flow velocity waveforms in normal and hypoxemic fetuses. *Am J Obstet Gynecol* **161**: 168–72.

21 Reuss ML, Rudolph AM. (1980) Distribution and recirculation of umbilical and systemic venous blood flow in fetal lambs during hypoxia. *J Devel Physiol* **2**: 71–84.

22 Behrman RE, Lees MH, Peterson EN, de Lannoy CW, Seeds AE. (1970) Distribution of the circulation in the normal and asphyxiated fetal primate. *Am J Obstet Gynecol* **108**: 956–69.

23 Edelstone DI, Rudolph AM, Heymann MA. (1980) Effects of hypoxemia and decreasing umbilical flow on liver and ductus venosus blood flows in fetal lambs. *Am J Physiol* **238**: H656–63.

24 Reuss ML, Rudolph AM, Dae MW. (1983) Phasic blood flow patterns in the superior and inferior venae cavae and umbilical vein of fetal sheep. *Am J Obstet Gynecol* **145**: 70–8.

25 Rizzo G, Arduini D, Romanini C. (1992) Umbilical vein pulsations: a physiologic finding in early gestation. *Am J Obstet Gynecol* **167**: 675–7.

26 Reed KL, Appleton CP, Anderson CF, Shenker L, Sahn DJ. (1990) Doppler studies of vena cava flows in human fetuses. Insights into normal and abnormal cardiac physiology. *Circulation* **81**: 498–505.

27 Indik JH, Chen V, Reed KL. (1991) Association of umbilical venous with inferior vena cava blood flow velocities. *Obstet Gynaecol* **77**: 551–7.

28 Nakai Y, Miyazaki Y, Matsuoka Y, Matsumoto M, Imanaka M, Ogita S. (1992) Pulsatile umbilical venous flow and its clinical significance. *Br J Obstet Gynaecol* **99**: 977–80.

29 Gudmundsson S, Huhta JC, Wood DC, Tulzer G, Cohen AW, Weiner S. (1991) Venous Doppler ultrasonography in the fetus with nonimmune hydrops. *Am J Obstet Gynecol* **164**: 33–7.

30 Rasanen J, Kirkinen P, Jouppila P. (1989) Right ventricular dysfunction in human fetal compromise. *Am J Obstet Gynecol* **161**: 136–40.

31 Rizzo G, Arduini D, Romanini C. (1992) Inferior vena cava flow velocity waveforms in appropriate- and small-for-gestational-age fetuses. *Am J Obstet Gynecol* **166**: 1271–80.

32 Arduini D, Rizzo G, Romanini C. (1993) The development of abnormal heart rate patterns after absent end-diastolic velocity in umbilical artery: analysis of risk factors. *Am J Obstet Gynecol* **168**: 43–50.

33 Indik JH, Reed KL. (1990) Variation and correlation in human fetal umbilical Doppler velocities with fetal breathing: evidence of the cardiac-placental connection. *Am J Obstet Gynecol* **163**: 1792–6.

34 Hecher K, Campbell S, Doyle P, Harrington K, Nicolaides K. (1994) Assessment of fetal compromise by Doppler ultrasound investigation of the fetal circulation. Arterial, intracardiac, and venous blood flow velocity studies. *Circulation,* in press.

35 Rightmire DL, Nicolaides KH, Rodeck CH, Campbell S. (1986) Midtrimester fetal blood flow velocities in rhesus isoimmunisation: relationship to gestational age and to fetal haematocrit in the untransfused patient. *Obstet Gynaecol* **21**: 233–6.

36 Nicolaides KH, Bilardo CM, Campbell S. (1990) Prediction of fetal anaemia by measurement of the mean blood velocity in the fetal aorta. *Am J Obstet Gynecol* **162**: 209–12.

37 Rizzo G, Nicolaides KH, Arduini D, Campbell S. (1990) Effects of intravascular fetal blood transfusion on fetal intracardiac Doppler velocity waveforms. *Am J Obstet Gynecol* **163**: 1231–8.

38 Mari G, Moise KJ, Deter RL *et al.* (1991) Doppler assessment of renal blood flow in the anemic fetus before and after intravascular transfusion for severe red cell alloimmunisation. *J Clin Ultrasound* **19**: 15–19.

CHAPTER 9

Colour Doppler imaging of the normal heart in healthy and complicated pregnancies

Ian Sullivan and Kevin Harrington

INTRODUCTION

The continuing improvement in both two-dimensional and Doppler ultrasound imaging has enabled echocardiography to play an increasing role in the structural and functional assessment of the fetal heart. Two-dimensional imaging of the four cardiac chambers and their connections is the essential step in assessing the structure of the normal fetal heart. Colour flow mapping, conventional spectral pulsed Doppler and M-mode echocardiography are adjuncts to the two-dimensional images and provide information about haemodynamic status and quantitative cardiac and great artery dimensions. Fetal echocardiography can be used in the detection of congenital heart defects (CHD), the assessment of arrhythmias and the functional assessment of the fetal heart in the presence of disease such as fetal hydrops.

This chapter will illustrate the normal heart and discuss the use of Doppler echocardiography in the compromised fetus. The use of Doppler ultrasound in the structurally abnormal heart is dealt with in Chapter 10.

THE FETAL CIRCULATION

The fetal circulation differs considerably from the postnatal circulation, principally because of the presence of the placenta and of non-inflated lungs (Fig. 9.1). Systemic venous return to the right atrium is a mixture of venous blood from the fetus (inferior and superior caval veins) and from the placenta (ductus venosus). The most oxygenated blood from the placenta is preferentially flow directed towards the foramen ovale by a flap of tissue in the right atrium (Eustachian valve). This ensures that the most oxygenated systemic venous blood is directed to the left ventricle and thence will be ejected into the ascending aorta towards the brain. Conversely, blood in the superior caval vein is preferentially directed to the tricuspid valve and right ventricle.

During ventricular systole blood from the right ventricle is ejected into the pulmonary trunk and while there is some flow directed to right and left pulmonary arteries, most of the ejected volume flows into the descending aorta via the arterial duct and thence to the placenta.

SCREENING FOR CONGENITAL HEART DEFECTS

Congenital anomalies of the heart are more common than anomalies of any other system, with almost 1% of liveborn infants affected. There is a wide variety of abnormalities, ranging from lesions which are likely to be lethal prenatally or in the immediate postnatal period, such as severe tricuspid valve abnormalities, to defects that may be asymptomatic and not noted until childhood or later, such as atrial septal defect.

Fetal echocardiography was initially validated in pregnancies at high risk for the presence of CHD, principally those where there was a family history of CHD or because extracardiac fetal anomalies had been detected. A family history of CHD confers increased risk for recurrence. When a heart abnormality has occurred previously in a sibling, the risk of recurrence of CHD, not necessarily the same lesion, is usually about 2% but may be higher for recurrence of conditions such as conotruncal abnormalities or hypoplastic left heart syndrome. The risk may be higher, up to 10% or more, when a parent is affected.[1] This is becoming increasingly relevant, as more survivors of surgery in infancy or early childhood for otherwise lethal cardiac defects are now approaching childbearing age.

There is also a high incidence of CHD in the fetus with an abnormal karyotype; for example, approximately 40% of liveborn infants with Down's syndrome have CHD, most typically atrioventricular septal defect. Hence, detection of fetal CHD may be a marker for abnormal karyotype. Heart abnormalities may also occur in association with other structural abnormal-

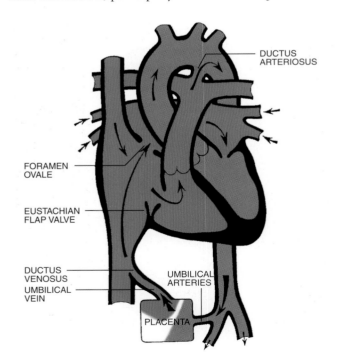

Fig. 9.1
Diagrammatic representation of the fetal circulation; red is venous blood, blue is arterial blood.

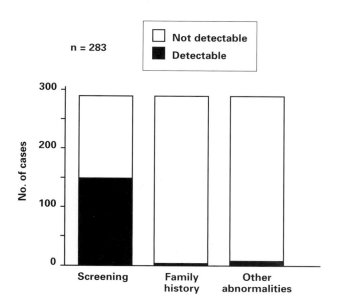

Fig. 9.2
The proportion of cases of severe congenital heart defects currently seen in infancy which would be detectable by using the four chamber view of the fetal heart as part of a population screening programme, compared to strategies entailing detailed assessment of the fetal heart in high risk pregnancies (those with a family history of congenital heart disease or those in whom an extracardiac abnormality is detected on fetal ultrasound. From reference 3.

ities detectable on fetal ultrasound assessment, such as omphalocele or renal abnormalities, and assessment of the fetal heart is important in determining the prognosis in the fetus in whom extracardiac abnormalities have been identified.

However, most liveborn infants with CHD are products of pregnancies without any known high-risk features. An increasing number of cases of CHD detected prenatally are referred for detailed fetal echocardiography because an abnormality of the fetal heart is suspected on routine ultrasound scan. The feasibility of a population based screening programme to detect cardiac abnormalities using a single four chamber view of the fetal heart was demonstrated in a prospective study in which only 21% of cardiac lesions associated with an abnormality of the four chamber view were overlooked.[2]

However, even in the highly motivated obstetric units participating in that study, the positive predictive value of a suspected cardiac abnormality was only 36%, so that more than half of suspected cardiac abnormalities were false positives and the fetal heart was actually normal. This emphasizes the importance of referring suspected cardiac abnormalities for detailed evaluation of the fetal heart. If effective four chamber view screen-

ing was applied to the whole population, about half of all severe cardiac defects currently seen in United Kingdom liveborn infants would be potentially detectable.[3] This represents a far greater yield than the proportion of cardiac defects that can be detected if detailed fetal echocardiography is restricted to high risk pregnancies (Fig. 9.2).

IMAGING THE FETAL HEART

The main prerequisite for fetal echocardiography is the ability to obtain clear images of the heart, with consistent planes of insonation to minimize the misinterpretation of artefact. It is possible to evaluate fetal cardiac connections from about 14–15 weeks' gestation by conventional transabdominal fetal echocardiography in some subjects, but more reliable images of the fetal heart are obtained in the majority of pregnancies at about 18 weeks' gestation.[2] At this gestational age, the fetal spine and ribs have not calcified and unfavourable fetal lies are not usually persistent.

The four chamber view of the fetal heart is the cornerstone for recognition of structural heart disease (Fig. 9.3). The large liver pushes the cardiac apex in a cephalad direction so that the fetal heart has a much more horizontal orientation than in postnatal life. Conveniently, therefore, the four chamber view of the fetal heart is obtained by imaging a transverse section

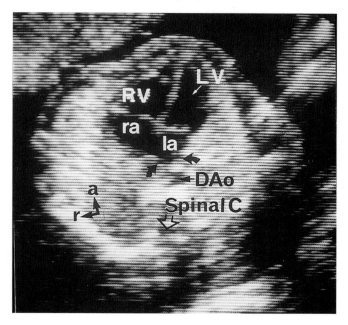

Fig. 9.3
The normal four chamber view of the fetal heart, a = anterior; DAo = descending aorta; la = left atrium; LV = left ventricle; r = right; ra = right atrium; RV = right ventricle; Spinal C = spinal cord; curved arrows indicate pulmonary veins.

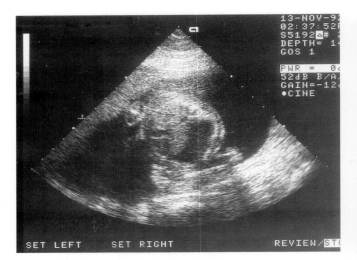

Fig. 9.4
The fetal is deviated into the right hemithorax by the presence of a large left pleural effusion

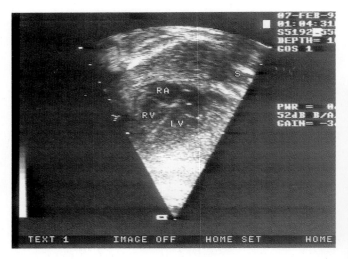

Fig. 9.5
Four chamber view of the fetal heart shows tissue at the margins of the foramen ovale billowing into the left atrium

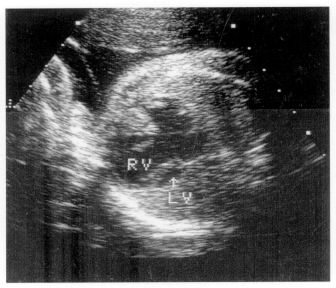

Fig. 9.6
Transverse section through the fetal thorax demonstrating cardiomegaly, right atrial and right ventricular disproportion and a common atrioventricular valve orifice. This is a heart with a complete atrioventricular septal defect and a hypoplastic left ventricle.

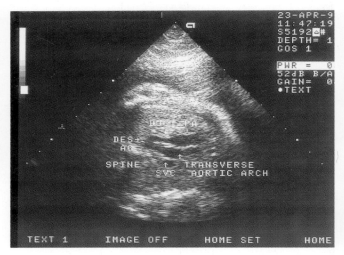

Fig. 9.7
Transverse section through the fetal thorax at a level slightly cephalad to the four chamber view. The pulmonary trunk continues as the arterial duct into the descending aorta. The transverse part of the aortic arch has a parallel orientation.

through the fetal thorax. This image cannot be duplicated postnatally, the closest equivalent being the apical four chamber view in which the scanning plane is in a line approximately joining left shoulder and right hip. It is easy to misinterpret an oblique four chamber fetal view, so that the inclusion of the longitudinal section of a least one rib is important to ensure that the imaging plane is transverse. The spine is used as the reference point for orientation.

There are several points that should be recognized from the normal four chamber view at 18–20 weeks' gestation.[4] The fetal heart area is not more than one-third of the area of the transverse section of the fetal thorax (Fig. 9.3). These relative areas can be measured easily by planimetry on most modern ultrasound machines. The cardiac apex is directed to the left but the normal heart is a relatively midline structure (compare Figs 9.3 and 9.4). The two atria are of similar size and the left atrium is closest to the spine. The descending aorta is adjacent to the posterior wall of the left atrium, just at the left of the spine. The two ventricles are of similar cavity size and wall thickness and have similar contraction.

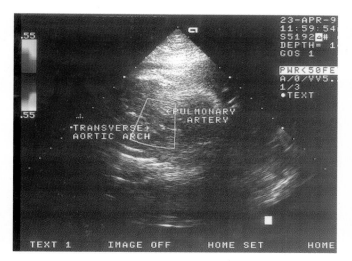

Fig. 9.8
Same fetus as Fig. 9.7. there are parallel streams of arterial blood flow in pulmonary trunk and transverse aortic arch.

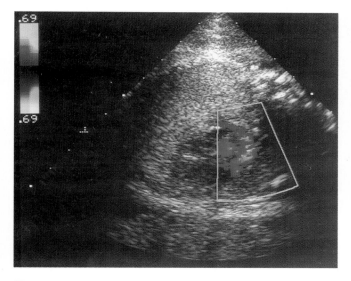

Fig. 9.9
Colour flow map demonstrating flow from the pulmonary trunk continuing into right pulmonary artery which passes posterior to the ascending aorta. The circular area of colour flow map is flow in the proximal part of the ascending aorta.

There are two separate atrioventricular valves which meet where the atrial septum joins the ventricular septum to form an offset cross. This occurs because the septal attachment of the tricuspid valve is positioned slightly more towards the cardiac apex than that of the mitral valve. Many other more subtle features may also be evident. The tissue at the margins of the foramen ovale billows into the left atrium, indicative of flow from right atrium to left atrium (Fig. 9.5). The right and left pulmonary veins more or less straddle the descending aorta as they drain into the back of the left atrium (see Fig. 9.3). A characteristic ridge of

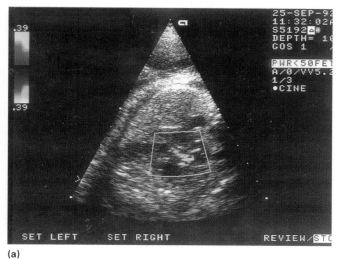

(a)

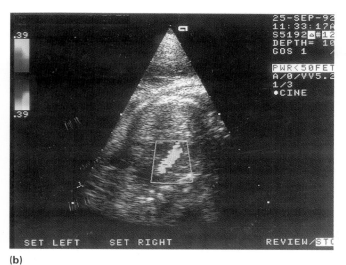

(b)

Fig. 9.10
Sections from the same fetus showing flow in (a) ascending aorta and (b) pulmonary trunk. The proximal great arteries cross over each other.

myocardium near the ventricular apex known as the moderator band identifies the morphologic right ventricle (see Fig. 9.3).

From the four chamber view alone, cardiac abnormalities characterized by cardiomegaly, atrial or ventricular cavity disproportion or abnormalities of the atrioventricular junction are evident (Fig. 9.6). These account for about 50% of severe congenital heart abnormalities currently seen in liveborn infants.[3]

The base or arterial pole of the heart requires additional assessment. A slightly more cephalad transverse section of the thorax than the four chamber plane can identify the pulmonary trunk in longitudinal section as it courses posteriorly from the right ventricular outflow tract, continuing as the arterial duct to join the descending aorta just to the left of the spine. The

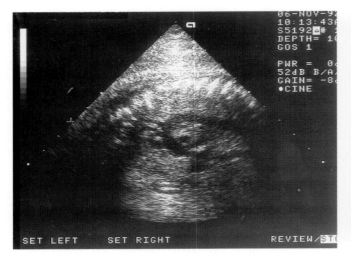

(a)

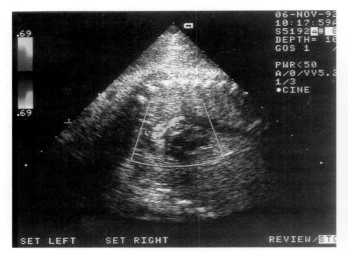

(b)

Fig. 9.11
Longitudal view of the aortic arch showing origin of the head and neck vessels (a) and the corresponding colour flow map (b)

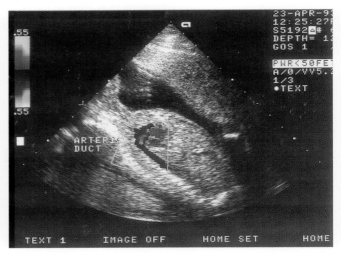

Fig. 9.12
Longitudal view of the ductal arch. The colour flow map demonstrates laminar flow passing from the pulmonary trunk into the descending aorta.

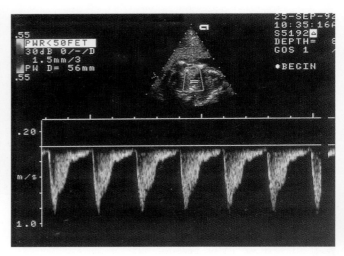

Fig. 9.13
Spectral Doppler display from arterial duct. A crisp Doppler signal is obtained despite poor views of the vessel which in this orientation has its longitudinal plane in the axial plane of the ultrasound beam.

transverse part of the aortic arch is adjacent to the distal part of the pulmonary trunk and the arterial duct, giving rise to two streams of parallel arterial blood flow (Figs 9.7 and 9.8). Tilting the transducer slightly in a caudal direction should enable the right pulmonary artery to be seen as it passes posterior to the ascending aorta (Fig. 9.9).

The ascending aorta arises from the left ventricular outflow tract and the first part of its course is directed towards the right shoulder, before it curves to become the transverse arch which, as noted above, is more or less parallel to the pulmonary trunk and arterial duct. Consequently, the proximal great arteries cross over each other (Fig. 9.10). The major relevance of this feature is that in hearts with ventriculoarterial discordance (transposed great arteries) and most forms of double outlet right ventricle, the proximal great arteries have a

parallel orientation. In the normal fetal heart, the pulmonary trunk is of slightly larger calibre than the ascending aorta. Longitudinal views of the aortic and ductal arches (Figs 9.11 and 9.12) are more difficult to obtain reliably in all studies. In order to screen for structural heart abnormalities most evaluation can be qualitative but when there is doubt about cardiac structure or performance, quantitative assessment of cardiac area, cavity dimensions or great artery size is necessary.

Colour flow Doppler has an important role to play in fetal echocardiography, but because much higher ultrasound energy is transmitted for pulsed Doppler interrogation compared to two-dimensional imaging,

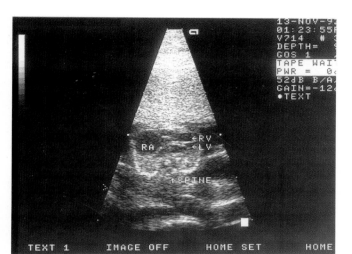

(a)

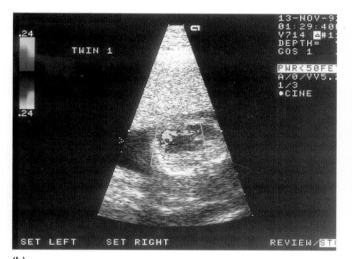

(b)

Fig. 9.14
Transverse views of the fetal thorax. (a) There is marked cardiomegaly, principally because of massive enlargement of right atrium. (b) Colour flow mapping demonstrates severe tricuspid regurgitation with turbulent flow seen passing from right ventricle to right atrium.

colour flow mapping should be used sparingly with low transmitted power setting.

The most common valuable role of colour flow mapping in fetal echocardiography is probably to confirm normal flow, especially in the great arteries in subjects in whom high quality two-dimensional images are hard to acquire, usually because of fetal lie or maternal obesity. This is particularly so when the long axis of a vessel is in the axial plane of the ultrasound beam. In this situation two-dimensional images are often much less clear than when the long axis of the vessel is at right angles to the axial plane of the ultrasound beam, but the vessel is in the optimal orientation for acquisition of colour flow and conventional spectral pulsed Doppler information (Fig. 9.13).

Colour flow signals identify sites of laminar or disturbed flow and facilitate optimal alignment of the sample volume for quantitative pulsed Doppler assessment. Colour flow may be helpful in some circumstances in confirming pulmonary venous flow to the left atrium (see below), demonstrating flow variation at the foramen ovale, and is extremely sensitive in detecting valvar regurgitation (Fig. 9.14).

PITFALLS IN FETAL ECHOCARDIOGRAPHY

The normal fetal circulation includes non-restrictive communications between right atrium and left atrium

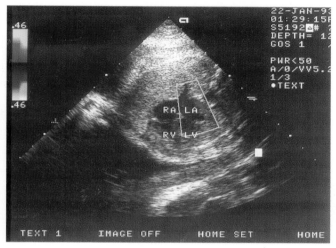

Fig. 9.15
Colour flow map demonstrating flow from right to left pulmonary veins to left atrium.

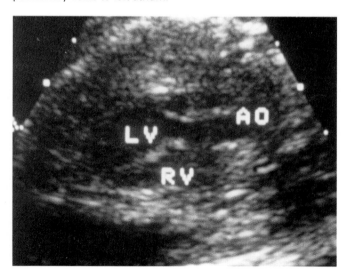

Fig. 9.16
Large subaortic VSD. The ascending aorta overrides the trabecular spetum. These is no ventricular disproportion evident.

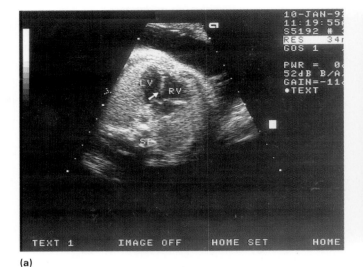

(a)

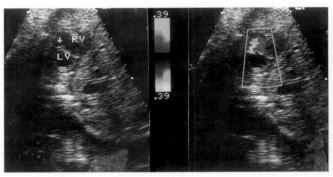

(b)

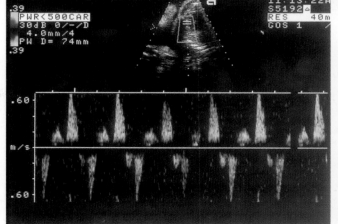

(c)

Fig. 9.17

(a) Obliqued four chamber view shows a possible apical VSD (small arrow). (b) The apparent VSD appears larger when the scanning plane is adjusted so that the muscular septum is at right angles to the scanning plane, and colour flow mapping confirms flow between left ventricle and right ventricle at this site. (c) Spectral analysis of VSD flow shows bidirectional flow at low velocity.

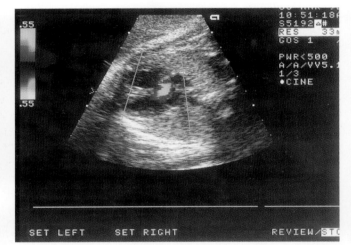

(a)

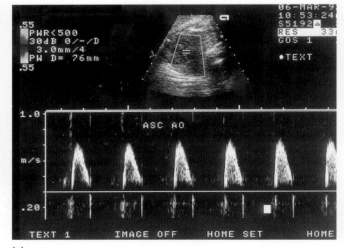

(b)

(c)

Fig. 9.18

(a) Long axis view of normal left ventricular outflow tract. (b) Colour flow mapping in the left ventricular outflow tract. (c) Pulsed Doppler spectral signal from this site.

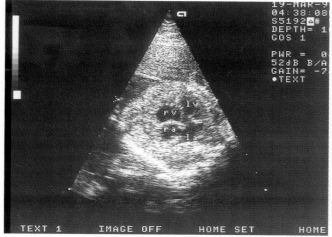

(a)

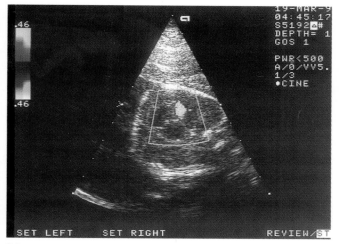

(b)

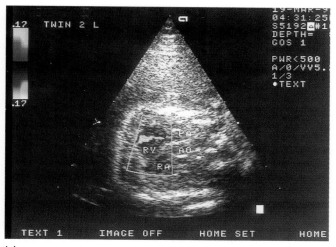

(c)

Fig. 9.19
Views of the heart in this fetus with a poorly compliant right ventricle demonstrate cardiomegaly, with (a) failure of the tricuspid valve to open in diastole. (b) Diastolic flow to the left ventricle appears normal, but there is no evidence of any inflow to the right ventricle. (c) Angling the transducer shows that the right ventricle fills in diastole by regurgitation through the pulmonary valve. There was retrograde flow in the pulmonary trunk.

(see Fig. 9.5) and pulmonary trunk and descending aorta (see Fig. 9.12). It is not possible to predict persistent patency of the arterial duct postnatally or the presence of a secundum ASD (atrial septal defect at the foramen ovale) unless perhaps it is very large.

Screening for structural heart abnormalities using the four chamber view can overlook important abnormalities of the arterial pole of the heart which have relatively normal four chamber appearances, such as tetralogy of Fallot or complete transposition of the great arteries. Right ventricular dominance becomes evident in normal pregnancies beyond about 28 weeks' gestation, but subtle degrees of this may be indicative of significant structural abnormalities such as coarctation of the aorta or total anomalous pulmonary venous connection in earlier pregnancy. There is usually hypoplasia of the transverse arch in isolated coarctation of the aorta and colour flow demonstration of pulmonary venous flow to the left atrium (Fig. 9.15) is helpful in excluding the latter diagnosis.

Ventricular septal defects (VSD) may not be obvious as there will be no major ventricular disproportion even in the presence of a large isolated VSD (Fig. 9.16). The balanced ventricular pressures means there is unlikely to be turbulent flow disturbance at the site of a VSD, but colour flow mapping may be very useful in confirming or refuting the presence of a suspected VSD (Fig. 9.17). Conversely, it is easy to obtain the misleading impression of a perimembranous or subaortic VSD when the imaging plane is tilted slightly cephalad from the four chamber view. This occurs because the normal left ventricular outflow tract is curved and the ventricular septum is thinnest at its membranous portion which is adjacent to the aortic valve in the normal heart. Ultrasound 'drop out' from this area of the septum may mean that the normally oriented ascending aorta appears to override the ventricular septum. If there is doubt, a two-dimensional view in the long axis of the left ventricle (Fig. 9.18) should be obtained to exclude an overriding aorta, but colour flow Doppler can be

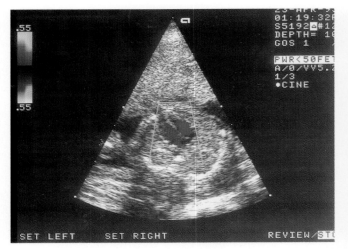

(a)

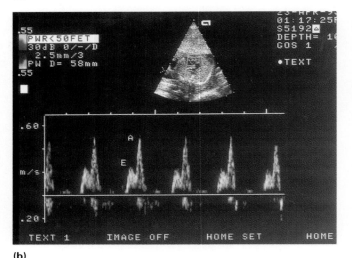

(b)

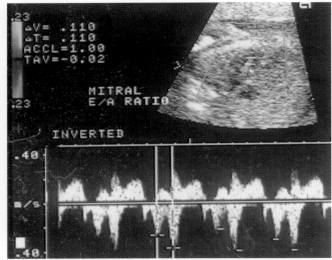

(c)

Fig. 9.20

(a) Four chamber view in diastole shows filling of both ventricles. (b) Pulsed Doppler spectral analysis of left ventricular filling demonstrates that late filling velocity coincident with atrial systole (A-wave) is of faster velocity than early diastolic filling (E-wave). This is the reverse of the ventricular filling pattern normally seen postnatally. (c) Variation in E/A ratio in a normal fetus.

also helpful in either confirming or refuting this diagnosis by demonstrating flow from both left and right ventricles entering the ascending aorta or normal left ventricular outflow tract flow respectively.

FETAL CARDIAC FLOW PATTERNS

The heart is the energy source for fetal arterial and venous flow so that flow patterns within the heart (e.g. abnormal ventricular proportions, valvar regurgitation) and cardiac contractile function should be considered when these are assessed (Fig. 9.19). Estimation of the actual volume of blood flow in vessels is difficult and prone to large error. To combat this, indices derived from the flow velocity waveform, such as the pulsatility index (PI), and individual velocity measurements have been found useful in assessing cardiac function and related changes in peripheral resistance.[5, 6]

In the fetus, flow across each atrioventricular valve (Fig. 9.20) is consistently greater during atrial contrac-

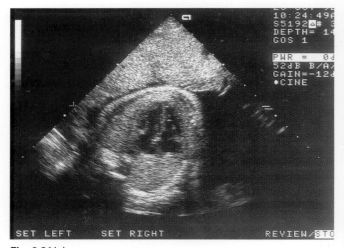

Fig. 9.21(a)

tion (A-wave) than during rapid ventricular filling (E-wave). This is the opposite to findings in the adult normal heart.[7] In the fetus the E/A ratios across the mitral

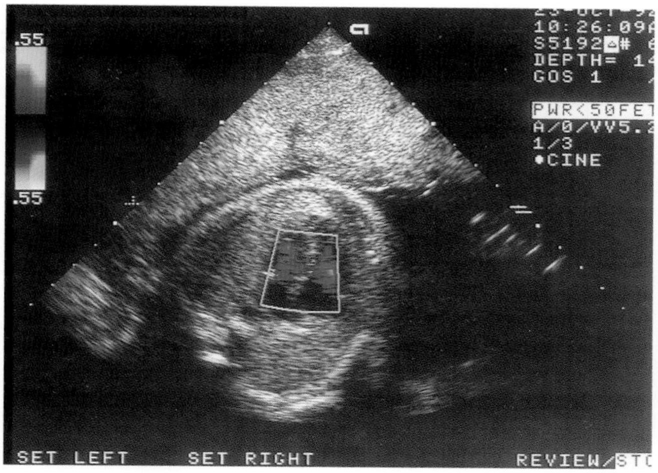

(b)

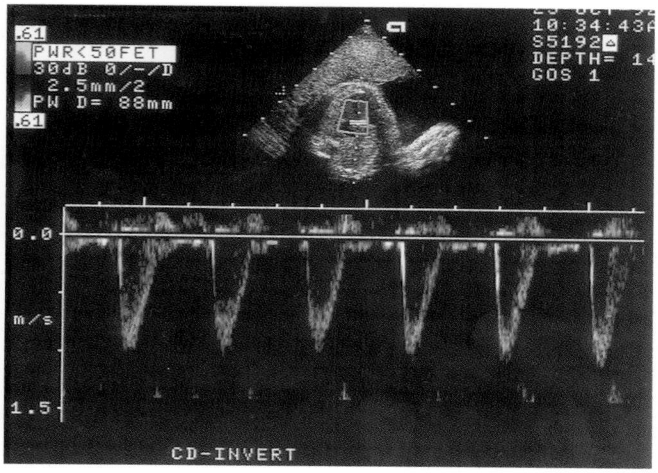

(e)

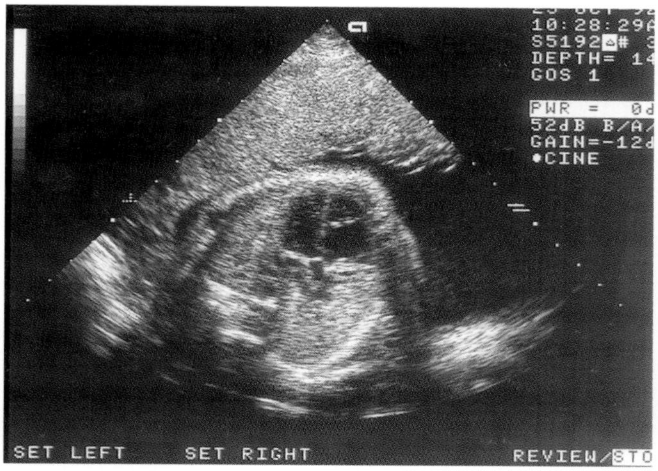

(c)

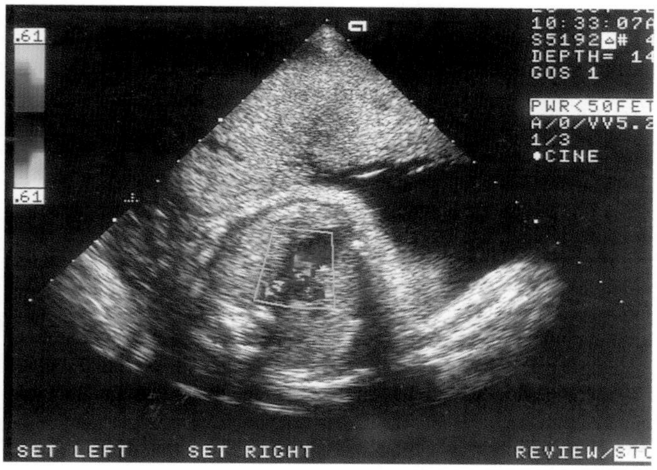

(f)

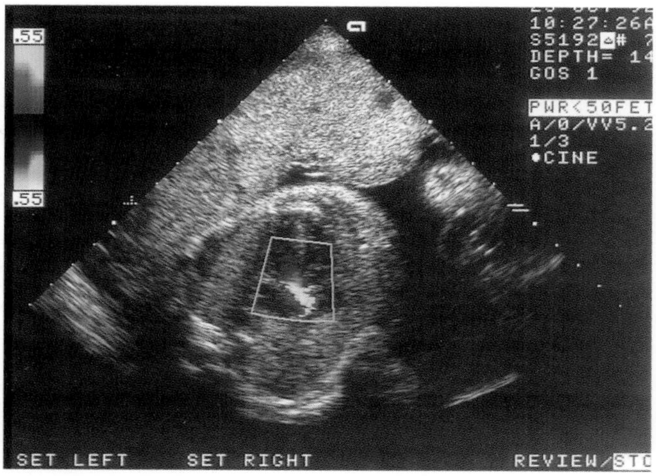

(d)

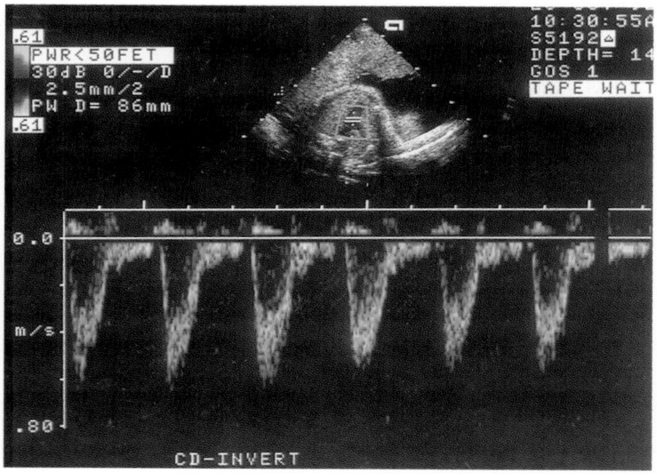

(g)

Fig. 9.21

(a) Four chamber view of the fetal heart in diastole. (b) Normal diastolic filling. (c) Tilting the transducer slightly cephalad shows left ventricular outflow tract and aorta with (d) colour flow signal in the ascending aorta, and (e) pulsed Doppler spectral signal from this site. (f) The right ventricular outflow tract and proximal pulmonary trunk crosses over the ascending aorta flow, with (g) pulsed Doppler spectral analysis from this site.

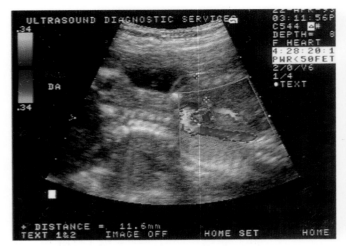

(a)

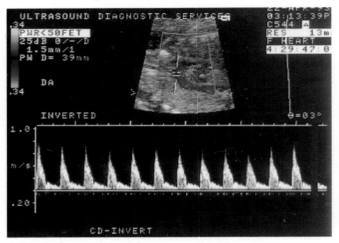

(b)

Fig. 9.22
(a) Longitudal view of the ductal arch with (b) pulsed Doppler interrogation of flow at the level of the duct

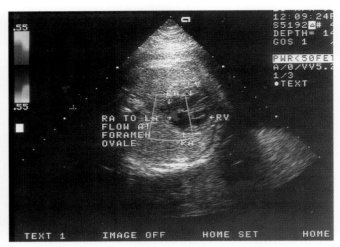

Fig. 9.23
Four chamber view with colour flow signal demonstrating flow from right atrium to left atrium at the foramen ovale.

and tricuspid valves are similar and velocities tend to increase from 20 weeks to term.[8] The atrio-ventricular flow velocities are heart rate dependent[9] and, in our experience, the great physiologic variability in fetal E/A ratios minimizes their value in fetal cardiac assessment (Fig. 9.20c). Doppler ultrasound allows estimation of blood flow through the inflow and outflow tracts of each cardiac ventricle, and the inflow (Fig. 9.21).[8] In the fetal heart right ventricular stroke volume normally exceeds that of the left ventricle, indicating right ventricular dominance *in utero*.[9]

Systolic velocities in the ductus arteriosus are the highest blood flow velocities found in the fetal cardio-vascular system (Fig. 9.22). Ductal velocities, assessed by pulsed Doppler spectral interrogation, increase with advancing gestational age when compared to the main pulmonary arterial velocities, which suggests that mild

relative constriction of the ductus may occur.[10] This may also explain the finding that with certain fetal behavioural states blood flow through the foramen ovale increases,[11] perhaps to supply well oxygenated blood via the left ventricle to the fetal brain (Fig. 9.23).

In animal studies, where premature closure of the ductus arteriosus was artificially created, right ventricular dilatation and tricuspid regurgitation developed *in utero*[12] and in another study persistent pulmonary hypertension was noted in the newborn lamb after *in utero* closure of the ductus arteriosus.[13] Premature closure or constriction of the ductus arteriosus DA in the human fetus could explain some of the cardiac changes that have been noted in neonatal life, in particular persistent pulmonary hypertension found in relation to perinatal asphyxia, meconium aspiration and postmaturity.

The fetal venous circulation is discussed in detail in Chapter 7.

CARDIAC CIRCULATORY CHANGES IN DISEASE

The sequence of changes that occurs in the circulation of the fetus exposed to hypoxia is illustrated in Chapter 8.

The increase in cerebral flow combined with increased resistance in the descending aorta leads to left ventricular dominance. In asymmetrically growth retarded fetuses (<10th centile), the finding of left ventricular dominance and a reduced total cardiac output was associated with a very poor perinatal outcome[14] and in fetuses with evidence of growth retardation and fetal blood flow redistribution, measurement of ascending aortic and pulmonary velocities suggested left ventri-

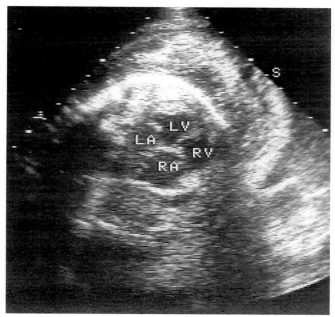

(a)

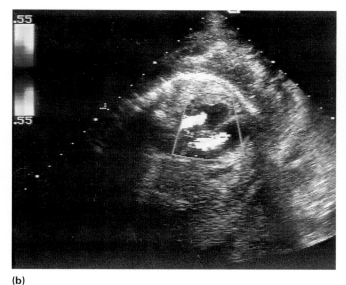

(b)

Fig. 9.24
Four chamber view in a hydropic fetus (a) shows cardiomegaly. Colour flow mapping (b) demonstrates severe regurgitation of both mitral and tricuspid valves. Contraction of both ventricles was also diminished.

cular dominance supporting this finding.[15]

Reverse blood flow in the inferior vena cava indicates that there is functional tricuspid incompetence. This can be assessed directly and may be seen as an early sign of right heart failure (Figs 9.24 and 9.25). An increase in the transverse diastolic diameter of the right ventricle and subsequently of the left ventricle seem to be early predictors of pathological fetal heart rate patterns in postdate pregnancies and this takes place before oligohydramnios is diagnosed.

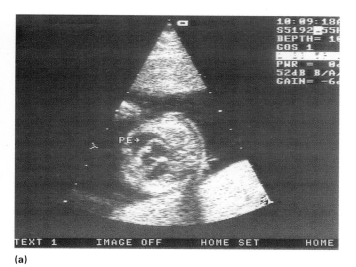

(a)

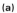

(b)

Fig. 9.25
Four chamber view in a hydropic fetus demonstrates mild cardiomegaly. (a) A pericardial effusion is evident, as well as (b) tricuspid regurgitation, demonstrated by turbulent colour flow in systole from right ventricle to right atrium.

The fetus with anaemia has a hyperdynamic circulation with velocities increased but resistance indices in the peripheral circulation relatively unchanged. As expected, there is a fall in fetal cardiac output after red cell transfusion.[15] Although useful in confirming the physiological changes that occur in the fetus, a clinical role for intracardiac Doppler in the assessment of the anaemic fetus has not yet been established.

ARRHYTHMIAS

Arrhythmias are an important cause of fetal heart failure. As noted above, ventricular filling in the fetus occurs predominantly in late diastole coincident with

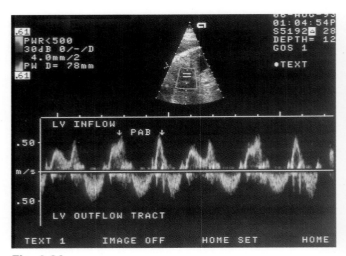

Fig. 9.26
Pulsed Doppler spectral signals obtained low in the left
ventricular outflow tract showing the sequence of normal
transmitral left ventricular filling. A sinus beat is followed by 2
premature atrial beats (PAB), then recurrence of the same
sequence followed by left ventricular ejection in the opposite
direction.

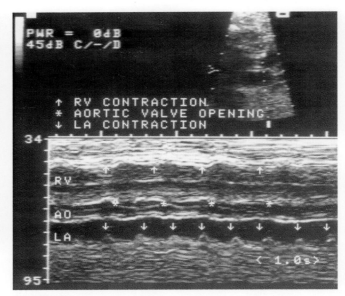

Fig. 9.27
Views from a fetus with complete heart block. The atrial rate is
about 150 beats/min estimated from atrial wall contraction,
whereas the ventricular rate is about 80/min. The ventricular
rate can be inferred from aortic valve opening, ventricular wall
contraction or from pulsed Doppler spectral signals in either
ventricular outflow tract.

atrial systole (see Fig. 9.20). The loss of atrial : ventricular synchrony is therefore likely to have worse
haemodynamic consequences for the fetus than is the
case postnatally, when ventricular filling occurs predominantly in early diastole.

The cardiac rhythm should be assessed in any
hydropic fetus, particularly as fetal tachycardia may be
amenable to drug therapy. Transient episodes of sinus
bradycardia are common in the midtrimester fetus and
transient episodes of sinus tachycardia with heart rate up
to about 180 beats/min become more common with
advance in pregnancy. Occasional premature beats are
also common in the normal fetus. However, sustained
tachycardia or bradycardia or persistent irregularity of
cardiac rhythm should be assessed in detail. Atrial depolarization can be inferred from atrial wall contraction and ventricular depolarization from ventricular
wall contraction or aortic valve opening.[16] However, it
is usually easier to confirm normal sinus rhythm by
placing the pulsed Doppler sample volume low in the
left ventricular outflow tract so that both inflow and
outflow spectral Doppler signals can be interrogated
(Fig. 9.26).

The most common cause of an irregular cardiac
rhythm is premature atrial beats; if these are conducted
to the ventricles, ventricular depolarization and ventricular contraction will occur earlier than would have
occurred in sinus rhythm. However, sufficiently premature atrial beats are typically not conducted to the
ventricles because the atrioventricular nodal conduction tissue is refractory, so that there is a delay before
the next ventricular contraction. If there are very fre-
quent premature atrial beats with blocked atrioventric-

ular conduction, there will be appreciable slowing of
the ventricular rate. Provided the heart is structurally
normal this is generally benign. However, premature
atrial beats may trigger supraventricular tachycardia in
susceptible individuals.

Complete heart block is characterized by bradycardia, with the rate of atrial contraction being greater
than the ventricular rate. It is important to exclude
structural heart disease such as left atrial isomerism or
congenitally corrected transposition of the great arteries in this situation. If the heart is structurally normal,
evidence of maternal connective tissue disease should
be sought. It is important not to misinterpret the slow
fetal heart rate as a sign of fetal distress during management of labour (Fig. 9.27).

Fetal tachycardia is usually the result of atrioventricular re-entry tachycardia (AVRT) or sometimes atrial
flutter. In AVRT, the re-entry circuit is completed by
an accessory pathway of conduction tissue between
atria and ventricles; this may be manifest as Wolff
Parkinson White syndrome with ventricular pre-
excitation on the surface electrocardiogram postnatally.
Atrial flutter may occur in the sick fetus with structural heart abnormality and AVRT may be associated
with specific abnormalities such as Ebstein's anomaly
of the tricuspid valve, but it is much more common for
the fetal heart to be structurally normal with these
arrhythmias. When atrial flutter is present, the atria
appear to 'quiver' in real-time imaging. Typically the
atrial rate is about 400/minute; 1:1 atrioventricular

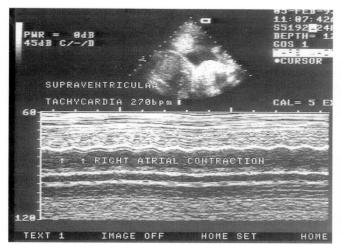

(a)

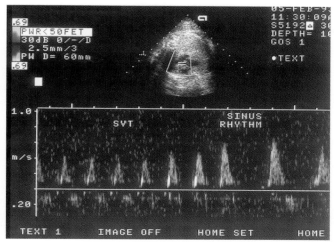

(c)

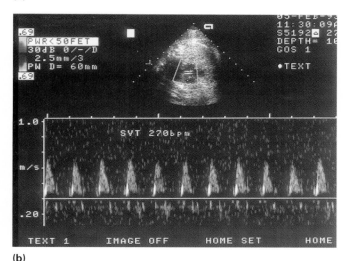

(b)

Fig. 9.28

Supraventricular tachycardia. (a) Both atrial and ventricular rates are 270 beats/min, as demonstrated by the rate of atrial wall contraction, and (b) the rate of the ventricular outflow tract spectral signal. (c) When spontaneous reversion to sinus rhythm occurs, there is not only reduction in ventricular rate but increase in flow velocity integral demonstrating improved stroke volume in sinus rhythm.

conduction is poorly tolerated at this rate and heart failure is likely. Fortunately there is often atrioventricular block present, which is usually 2:1 so that the ventricular rate is about 200/min which may be well tolerated. AVRT is characterized by a 1:1 atrioventricular relationship with ventricular rate usually 200–300/min (Fig. 9.28).

Therapy for supraventricular tachycardia should be considered when sustained tachycardia is identified and is indicated if features of incipient or established fetal heart failure are present. If there is no major fetal haemodynamic compromise maternal digoxin therapy is probably the treatment of first choice, although large maternal doses are needed to obtain adequate fetal blood levels. The tachyarrhythmia is life-threatening in the hydropic fetus and more aggressive antiarrhythmic drug treatment is justified. Flecainide is probably the treatment of first choice and early experience with this agent in the hydropic fetus with supraventricular tachycardia has been encouraging.[17]

SUMMARY

Screening for congenital heart disease has become accessible to most units performing obstetric ultrasound. The anatomy and function of the normal heart should be appreciated before attempting to diagnose congenital heart disease antenatally. If a structural lesion is suspected an expert opinion should be obtained before acting on the information. Detailed fetal echocardiography should also be considered in any pregnancy where there is a family history of congenital heart disease, extracardiac abnormalities have been detected or a chromosome abnormality is suspected.

Assessment of the fetal heart may also be important in the management of the compromized fetus. Colour and pulsed Doppler are probably unnecessary for screening purposes, but can be of enormous benefit in confirming normality and in the assessment of abnormal physiology.

REFERENCES

1 Whittemore R, Hobbins JC, Engle MA. (1982) Pregnancy and its outcome in women with and without surgical treatment of congenital heart disease. *Am J Cardiol* **50**: 361–70.

2 Sharland GK, Allan LD. (1992) Screening for congenital heart disease prenatally. Results of a 2½ year study in the South East Thames region. *Br J Obstet Gynaecol* **99**: 220–5.

3 Cullen S, Sharland G, Allan LD, Sullivan ID. (1992) Potential impact of population screening for prenatal diagnosis of congenital heart disease. *Arch Dis Child* **67**: 775–8.

4 Allan LD. (1989) Diagnosis of fetal cardiac abnormalities. *Arch Dis Child* **64**: 964–8.

5 Wladimiroff JW, Van den Wijngaard J, Degani S *et al.* (1987) Cerebral and umbilical arterial blood flow velocity waveforms in normal and growth-retarded pregnancies. *Obstet Gynaecol* **69**: 705–9.

6 Al-Ghazali W, Chita SK, Chapman MG, Allan LD. (1989) Evidence of redistribution of cardiac output in asymmetrical growth retardation. *Br J Obstet Gynaecol* **96**: 697–704.

7 Reed KL, Sahn DJ, Scagnelli S *et al.* (1986) Doppler echocardiographic studies of diastolic function in the human fetal heart: changes during gestation. *J Am Coll Cardiol* **8**: 391–5.

8 Kenny JF, Plappert T, Doubilet P *et al.* (1986) Changes in intracardiac blood flow velocities and right and left ventricular stroke volumes with gestational age in the normal human fetus: a prospective Doppler echocardiographic study. *Circulation* **74**: 1208–16.

9 Van der Mooren K, Barendregt LG, Wladimiroff JW. (1991) Fetal atrioventricular and outflow tract flow velocity waveforms during normal second half of pregnancy. *Am J Obstet Gynecol* **165**: 668–74.

10 Huhta J, Moise KJ, Fisher DJ *et al.* (1987) Detection and quantitation of constriction of the fetal ductus arteriosus by Doppler echocardiography. *Circulation* **75**: 406–12.

11 van Eyck, Stewart P, Wladimiroff JW. (1990) Human fetal foramen ovale waveforms relative to behavioural states in normal term pregnancy. *Am J Obstet Gynecol* **163**: 1239–42.

12 Tulzer G, Gudmundsson S, Rotondo KM *et al.* (1991) Acute fetal ductal occlusion in lambs. *Am J Obstet Gynecol* **165**: 775–8.

13 Morin FC. (1989) Ligating the ductus arteriosus before birth causes persistent pulmonary hypertension in the newborn lamb. *Pediatr Res* **25**: 245–50.

14 Al-Ghazali W, Chapman MG, Allan LD. (1988) Doppler assessment of the cardiac and uteroplacen tal circulations in normal and complicated pregnancies. *Br J Obstet Gynaecol* **95**: 575–80.

15 Rizzo G, Nicolaides KH, Arduini D, Campbell S. (1990) Effects of intravascular fetal blood transfusion on fetal intracardiac Doppler velocity waveforms. *Am J Obstet Gynecol* **163**: 1231–8.

16 Allan LD, Anderson RH, Sullivan ID, Campbell S, Holt D, Tynan M. (1983) Evaluation of fetal arrhythmias by echocardiography. *Br Heart J* **50**: 240–5.

17 Allan LD, Chita SK, Sharland GK, Maxwell D, Priestly K. (1991) Flecainide in the treatment of fetal tachycardias. *Br Heart J* **65**: 46–8.

CHAPTER 10

Fetal colour Doppler imaging in congenital heart diseases

Laurent Fermont and Jérôme Le Bidois

INTRODUCTION

In the last decade fetal echocardiography has enabled the prenatal detection of congenital heart diseases. With close collaboration between obstetricians and paediatric cardiologists, this new field has become established as an essential part of the practice of fetal medicine. The aim of fetal cardiology is to detect as accurately as possible the major anatomic or haemodynamic anomalies that predispose the fetus (and eventually the child) to the consequences of the functional problems that may ensue, and to help in identifying the fetus that may have a cardiac lesion as part of a wider problem, e.g. Down's syndrome.

It is possible with high-resolution two-dimensional echocardiography to diagnose most of the major anomalies. However, the anatomic lesion is only one aspect of the cardiac disease. Parents faced with the diagnosis of a congenital heart lesion in their prospective child are naturally concerned as to the wider consequences of the worrying situation in which they find themselves. It is often the case that the life of the fetus or neonate is not immediately threatened because of the lesion or its haemodynamic effects. The concerns of parents not only relate to this immediate situation, but also to the duration and quality of this future life, with or without surgery.

Therefore, establishing a diagnosis prenatally is not enough. It is of paramount importance to discuss the physiological consequences of the diagnosis, the feasibility of surgical procedures, and the prospect of the fetus being able to eventually have a 'normal' quality of life. These goals can be initially achieved with detailed examination of the fetal cardiac anatomy, through understanding the evolution of the functional changes in the circulation, and by complementing the anatomical data with haemodynamic studies.

Developments in physiological assessment of the different components of the cardiovascular system has become possible with the introduction of duplex systems (Doppler ultrasound combined with B-mode imaging in one transducer/machine), known as 2D echodoppler. Even with this advance there were difficulties with pulsed Doppler examination of the fetal heart, especially with an active fetus and a complex lesion. It is only since the arrival with colour flow Doppler imaging the difficulties with continuous and range-gated pulsed Doppler examination has been overcome, and the potential for the widespread use of fetal echocardiography has begun to be realized.

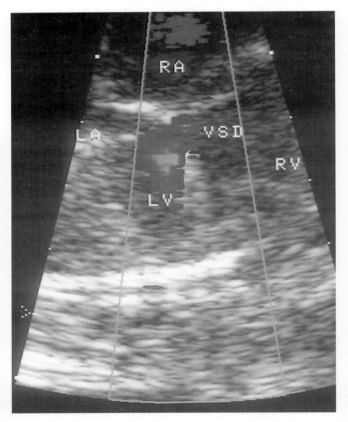

Fig. 10.2
Perimembraneous ventricular septal defect. The extent of flow across a perimembraneous defect and whether or not there are extensions to the inlet, can be assessed qualitatively with CDI. CDI can help in differentiating the type of VSD present, and associated lesions if present. Figs 10.3, 10.4 and 10.5 help to illustrate this point.

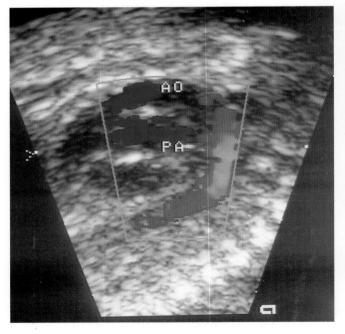

Fig. 10.1
Colour flow image of the great arteries. Colour Doppler imaging (CDI) can be helpful when there is poor visualization as a result of an unsatisfactory fetal lie.

The diagnosis of structural cardiac anomalies

Nearly all the significant congenital heart diseases are detectable with 2D echodoppler alone: the presence or absence of normal cardiac structural anatomy, the intracardiac structures, the assessment of any relative or absolute disproportion in the dimensions of the cardiac chambers and vessels, and any problems with the anatomical atrioventricular and ventriculo-arterial valves can be assessed without the use of Doppler ultrasound.

Colour Doppler echocardiography

Colour Doppler flow mapping is helpful in:

- establishing a definitive diagnosis when there is poor visualization, e.g. the great arteries (Fig. 10.1);
- obtaining more information where 2D echodoppler alone is often unable to provide a clear diagnosis;
- visualizing structures otherwise difficult to assess and to detect malformations otherwise missed;

- helping to diagnose unusual diseases in the fetus;
- determining the progression of a lesion diagnosed prenatally.

Differentiating simple and complicated ventricular septal defects

Colour Doppler flow mapping is helpful in establishing a definitive diagnosis when there is poor visualization, e.g. isolated ventricular septal defects (VSD), where colour flow mapping cannot only confirm the defect but also localize its position.

A VSD within the septum may be perimembranous with or without extensions to the inlet (Fig. 10.2) or the infundibular parts; alternatively there may be an inlet and atrioventricular lesion (Fig. 10.3), it may be trabeculated (Fig. 10.4) or the infundibular portion may be affected with or without septal malalignments (Fig. 10.5). Visualizing the ventricular septal defect precisely is also important in determining the prognosis for this and many other malformations.

The position and the number of the ventricular septal defects is also important: multiple trabeculated defects, inlet defects, and very large defects all carry a different prognosis regarding the results of postnatal surgical procedures. In complex malformations (such as arterial malpositions, univentricular hearts), it is partic-

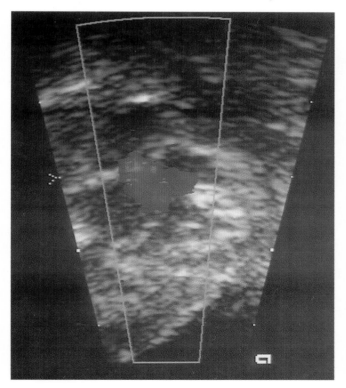

Fig. 10.3
Atrioventricular VSD. The full extent of this lesion can be appreciated when colour is applied. In addition to confirming the defect seen with real time imaging, the amount and direction of flow disturbance can be investigated.

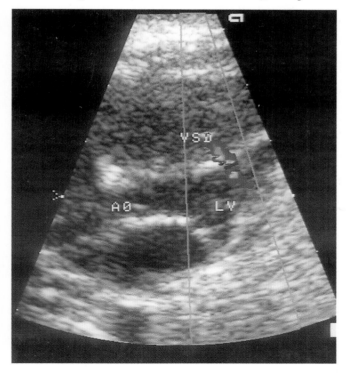

Fig. 10.4
The left ventricle and aortic outlet with a trabeculated VSD illustrated with CDI.

ularly important to study the size of the ventricular defects and their possible haemodynamic restrictions. Such restrictions could lead to hypoplasia of the contralateral ventricle (Fig. 10.6) with a hypoplastic vascular bed downstream. If the great arteries are in their normal position, a restrictive ventricular septal defect could lead to pulmonary hypoplasia creating further difficulties with postnatal surgery.

If there is a malposition of the arteries, a restrictive interventricular septal defect could lead to hypoplasia of the subaortic ventricle and, by extension, of the aortic arch. It is important to visualize the pulmonary artery, measure its size as well as anatomy, and consider its position in relation to the aorta and ventricles. This type of detailed examination is necessary for the diagnosis/exclusion of a malposition, pulmonary atresia with ventricular septal defect, Fallot's tetralogy or truncus arteriosus (Fig. 10.7).

Venous drainage to the heart

Colour Doppler is useful in the detection of lesions in the systemic venous collecting system, especially as the various vessels converge on the right atrium, the inferior vena cava, the hemiazygos continuation, the superior vena cava, the persistent left vena cava (to

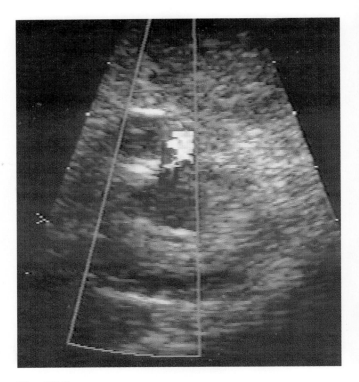

Fig. 10.6
VSD with hypoplasia of the contralateral ventricle. If the position of the great arteries is normal, a restrictive ventricular septal defect could lead to pulmonary hypoplasia creating further diffioculties for postnatal surgery

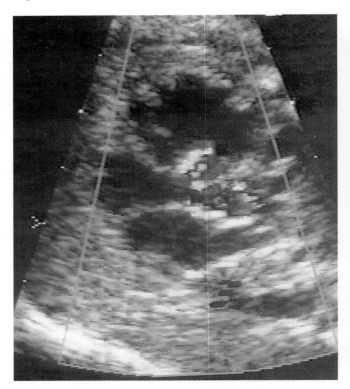

Fig. 10.5
Abnormally positioned septum with a VSD clearly shown as flow towards the transducer (red)

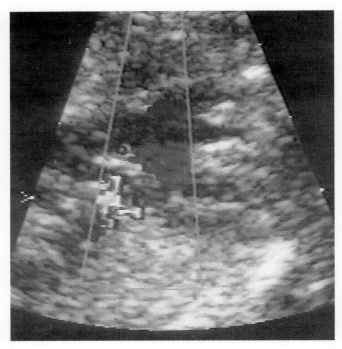

Fig. 10.7
A large VSD with overriding pulmonary artery. Detailed examination is required to diagnose/exclude malposition, pulmonary atresia with a VSD, Fallot's tetralogy or truncas arteriosus.

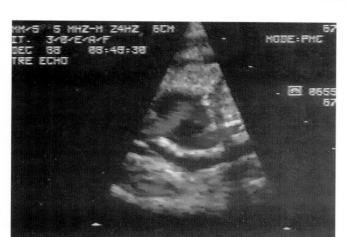

Fig. 10.8
Total anomalous pulmonary venous drainage. This condition does not affect cardiac function in fetal life, but creates a number of problems after birth, which may not be attributed to the lesion in the first instance. Antenatal detection is therefore important. In this image a large venous conduit or collector can be seen passing the left atrium with flow directed towards the liver. This type of anomalous drainage is most amenable to surgery.

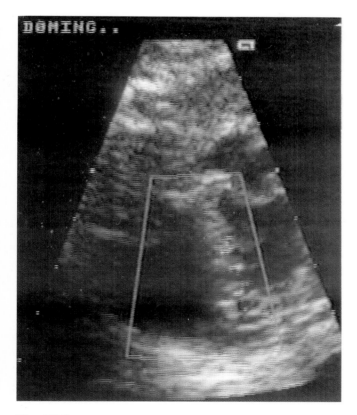

Fig. 10.9
Unusual and rare cardiac anomalies can be detected prenatally. Massive vascular dilatation of the pulmonary artery (absent pulmonary valve syndrome) with obstruction and insufficiency at the valvular level explains the findings in this fetus.

coronary sinus), the absent right vena cava, and the unroofed coronary sinus can all be visualized. These anomalies are sometimes isolated; they can also be associated with complex cardiac malformations and be of importance with regard to the definition of cardiac syndromes and for the purpose of prenatal surgical evaluation. Pulmonary venous return is also important in prenatal diagnosis. For example, it is important to localize the venous ostia as anomalies of pulmonary venous drainage can make some malformations very difficult to treat surgically (e.g. common atria). Visualizing the venous vasculature and flow through the foramen ovale is helpful when describing the atrio-ventricular connections. For instance if a ventriculo-arterial discordance (transposition of the great arteries) has been detected, with or without ventricular septal defect or pulmonary stenosis, it is important to exclude an associated atrioventricular defect, as this alters the prognosis, dividing the condition into the 'atrio-ventriculo and ventriculo-arterial' discordance ('anatomically corrected transposition of the great arteries').

Early detection of total anomalous pulmonary venous return is a challenge for neonatologists because this anomaly can lead to early severe haemodynamic failure. There is no impairment of haemodynamics during fetal life. Visualization of the venous drainage to the left atria is clearly improved by colour Doppler. Several anatomical 'miscellaneous' forms of pulmonary venous drainage have been described, but the lesion most amenable to the effects of surgery are those where a venous collector can be seen, passing behind the left atria with flow directed toward the liver through the diaphragm (Fig. 10.8) or via the superior vena cava. Intracardiac forms of the coronary sinus could be misinterpreted as a partial atrioventricular canal.

Unusual and uncommon fetal cardiac anomalies

Many congenital heart diseases are very rare, and are not usually identified until after birth; the reported cases are obviously rare before birth, raising the question as to their natural prenatal history. A massive vascular dilatation may be the enlarged pulmonary artery of an absent pulmonary valve syndrome with obstruction and insufficiency at the valvular level (Fig. 10.9); a 'pseudo-cyst' may be a false-aneurysm of the left ventricle (Fig. 10.10), a subaortic diastolic insufficiency responsible for a huge hypertrophy-dilatation of the left ventricle may be secondary to the very rare 'aorta-left ventricular tunnel'.

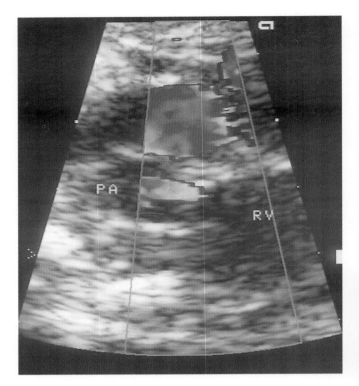

Fig. 10.10
A 'Pseudo-cyst' may be discovered to be a false-aneurysm of the left ventricle when flow is assessed with colour Doppler imaging

Monitoring the progression of an anomaly prenatally

The extra information obtained with colour Doppler imaging is important in helping to make a more accurate evaluation of the severity of a specific disease already diagnosed with conventional imaging. As many lesions that fall under the same umbrella can have differing outcomes, colour Doppler is also important in allowing individual patients to be followed up more precisely, with care being determined in part by the specifics of the lesion found.

THE DIAGNOSIS OF CARDIAC ANOMALIES WITH FLOW VELOCITY WAVEFORMS

Continuous wave (CW) and pulsed Doppler (PD) can be of value in certain circumstances when making a prenatal diagnosis of a cardiac lesion. Colour Doppler allows a more accurate placement of the PD range gate, thereby minimizing errors of interpretation, and improving the accuracy of the measurements. Colour Doppler, therefore, ensures the validity of the measurements by visualizing the direction of flow. The

information provided by flow velocity waveforms includes:

- velocity measurements, absolute and relative;
- pressure gradients between chambers and vessels;
- flow distribution;
- flow direction.

Flow velocity measurements

Defining direction of flow and calculating velocity allows an assessment of myocardial function and flow calculations. Colour Doppler/M-Mode studies provide time-related information, useful as soon as a leakage is detected (Fig. 10.11). Valvular insufficiencies can provide valuable information in case of ventricular dys-

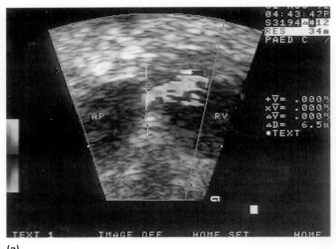

(a)

(b)

Fig. 10.11
Leakage from the pulmonary artery into the right ventricle through an incompetent pulmonary valve (a). M-mode/colour provides as assessment of the leakage throughout the cardiac cycle (b).

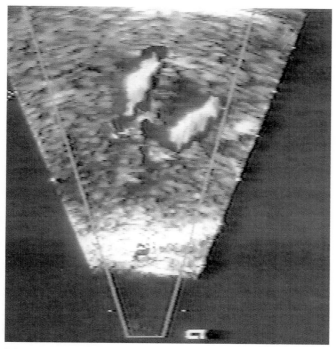

(a)

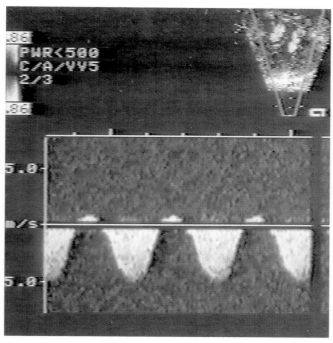

(b)

Fig. 10.12
Mitral insufficiency (a) with an abnormal flow velocity waveform (b) which in this case is associated with a left ventricular cardiomyopathy

function (right ventricle): fetal distress, iatrogenic aetiology, structural heart disease (left ventricle): left cardiomyopathy (Fig. 10.12), structural heart disease.

Pressure gradients

Pressure gradients can be measured across a localized stenosis by using the modified Bernouilli's equation and the maximal instantaneous velocity (Vmax) such that: Gradient (mmHg) $= 4 \,(Vmax)^2$. This formula has been validated after birth by neonatal haemodynamic studies. It has been tested in fetuses with cardiac diseases by prospective monitoring during follow-up and then compared with the results obtained at birth. Pressure gradient measurements can be obtained at the following sites:

PULMONARY AND AORTIC OUTFLOW TRACTS

Pressure gradients or truncal maximal pressure gradients (mean gradients when using mean velocities), can be measured in the pulmonary and aortic outflow tracts (Fig. 10.13). The results must be interpreted with caution. Small angle variations can result in significant differences in gradient evaluation. The results depend on the status of the fetal circulation (gestational age, ductal and isthmic status, descending aorta and placental haemodynamics). Therefore, by the time the

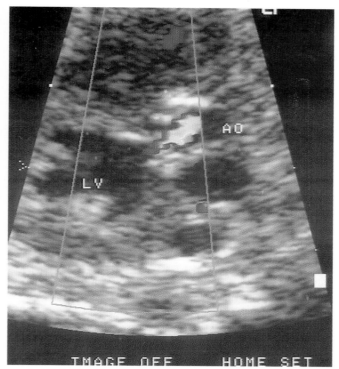

Fig. 10.13
It is possible to measure pressure gradients across the pulmonary and aortic (seen here) valves, which may be helpful in assessing a stenosis. Caution is advized when interpreting the results as a small change or error in the angle of insonation can lead to large degrees of error.

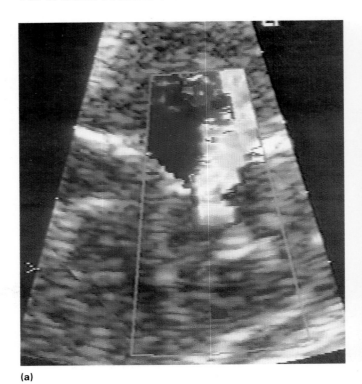

(a)

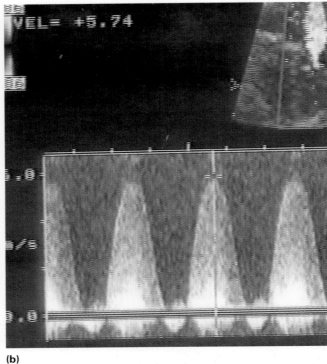

(b)

Fig. 10.14
Systolic colour (a) and flow velocity waveform (b) assessment. Calculation of maximum velocities (Vmax) allows an indirect calculation of ventricular pressures (assuming, in the absence of hydrops an atrial pressure of 5 mmHg). This investigation may be useful when there is any cause of increased ventricular pressure that requires more detailed investigation.

pressure gradient indicates a problem exists, there is often significant obstruction.

ATRIOVENTRICULAR INFLOW

Systolic pressure gradients can be measured at this level. In the absence of hydrops a right and left atrial pressure at 5 mmHg leads to an estimate of right or left systolic pressures according to the modified formula,

ventricular pressure (mmHg) =
$4(Vmax)^2$ + atrial pressure (Figs 10.12 and 10.14)

This information enables the measurement of elevated ventricular pressures in case of an outflow obstruction (aortic or pulmonary stenosis), ductal stenosis, coarctation of the aorta, or ventricular impairment. A comprehensive examination involves the study of stenotic atrioventricular valves including measurement of the mean diastolic pressure gradients, especially important at the mitral level, where stenotic anatomic anomalies are frequently associated with insufficiency. In aortic lesions, where the finding of mitral valve insufficiency is inconsistent and the haemodynamic variations at the ductal level can hinder proper evaluation of the pressure gradients, the measurements are mainly those of systolic pressure gradients at the outflow tract levels.

THE DUCTUS ARTERIOSUS

A stenosis of the ductus arteriosus can be secondary to indomethacin infusion. The anatomy of the pulmonary

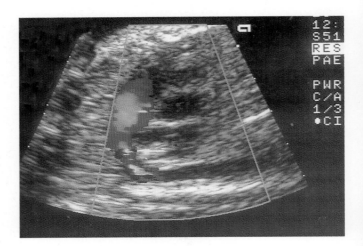

Fig. 10.15
Ductus arteriosus. CD imaging of the ductus often shows aliasing, as seen here. This reflects the relatively high velocities and mild turbulence in blood flow as it passes through the ductus

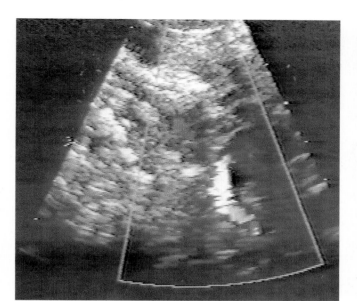

(a)

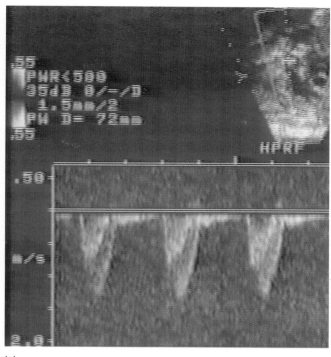

(c)

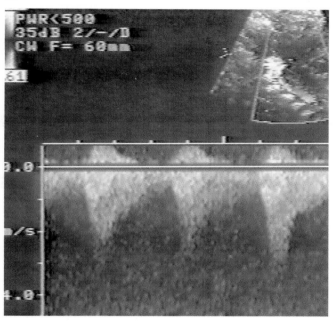

(b)

Fig. 10.16

(a) This image of the ductus arteriosus demonstrates the dramatic increase in maximum velocities that are seen in flow through this vessel. It is often the combination of aliasing and maximum velocities that help confirm that the ductus is being examined. (b) Flow velocity waveform of blood flow through the ductus arteriosus. The pressure gradient and amount of sytolic and diastolic flow can be assessed. (c) Indomethacin therapy is associated with premature closure of the ductus arteriosus. If therapy is discontinued the degree and change in the stenosis can be assessed with Doppler, as seen in this example.

artery is usually normal. Without colour Doppler, the diagnosis rests on imaging tricuspid insufficiency and the functional consequences of the stenosis in the right ventricle. Colour Doppler visualizes the flow at the ductus, which may be mildly turbulent (Fig. 10.15) or show dramatic increases in maximum velocities (Fig. 10.16a). With the transducer parallel to the ductal flow it is possible to measure pressure gradients and analyse the 'systolic/diastolic type' waveform (Fig. 10.16b). Monitoring the evolution of a stenosis is also possible, especially where the cause is drug related, and the drug is discontinued (Fig. 10.16c).

THE FORAMEN OVALE

The valve of the foramen ovale normally bulges toward the left atria, indicating the direction of the venous flow. Pulsed Doppler studies provide valuable information about the movements of the foramen ovale related to ventricular filling and atrial systole. The double-peaked diastolic waveform is normally low velocity. Colour Doppler improves the physiological understanding of changes in the flow patterns within the atria and through the valve. It visualizes changes of the non-restricted haemodynamics, allows measurement of the important diameters, as well

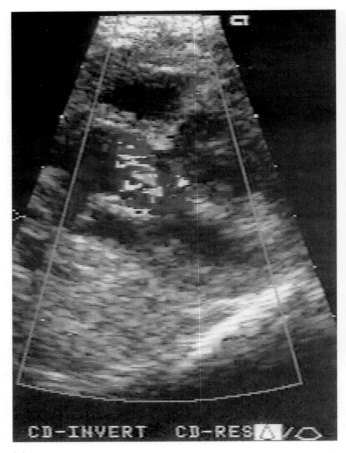

(a)

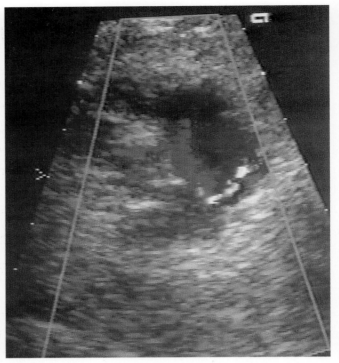

(b)

Fig. 10.17
(a) Transposition of the great arteries with restriction at the level of the foramen ovale (demonstrated by the colour flow aliasing seen this picture). (b) The same condition viewed from another angle.

as right atrial haemodynamics, looking for intra-atrial mixing of the inferior and superior caval returns.

The finding of a left-to-right shunt at high velocity suggests a restrictive foramen ovale (assessed by calculations from the Bernouilli's formula). This may be of value when diagnosing fetal diseases associated with hydrops, right ventricular impairment, right-left structural disproportions in diameter, ventricular dysfunction, arrhythmias and a wide range of congenital heart diseases. It occurs frequently in the case of left ventricular outflow tract obstructions and raises the question about it being responsible for the pathophysiological changes, perhaps as a 'trigger' and has led some cardiologists to consider the indication of a prenatal atrioseptostomy.

The diagnosis of a restrictive foramen ovale is especially useful if the haemodynamic status after birth depends on permeability. Because of its potential influence on perinatal management, it is important to detect restriction of the foramen ovale in specific diseases. The best example is the simple transposition of the great arteries with survival dependent on venous mixing at the atrial level; a restriction ends up in acute acidosis, which can be relieved by Rashkind's atrioseptostomy as an emergency procedure. Prenatal diagnosis of this lesion results in an immediate

infusion of prostaglandins after birth, with an immediate rather than delayed arterial switch operation (Fig. 10.17).

OTHER SITES

Calculations can be performed at every site within the cardiovascular system. The severity of distal vascular stenosis can be assessed in this way.

Analysis of the direction of flow

The distribution of the flow through the foramen ovale, the ductus arteriosus and the isthmus of the aorta can all be assessed.

ATRIOVENTRICULAR VALVES

Atrioventricular valve insufficiency allows the assessment of intraventricular pressures. Furthermore, it supports a positive diagnosis from a 2D-echo aspect of mitral or tricuspid malformation, which is sometimes difficult to establish. Tricuspid insufficiency is often secondary to functional causes. It is important to note that a mild leakage may occur in a normal heart. The diagnosis of mitral

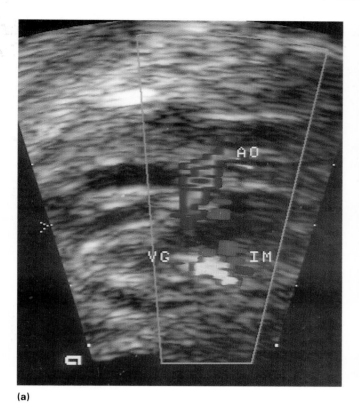

(a)

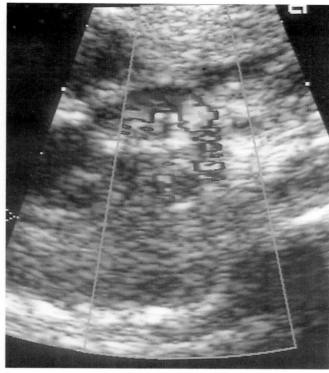

(b)

Fig. 10.18
Leakage through the atrioventricular valves is often associated with other anomalies, especially of the mitral valve is affected. In this example there is mitral insufficiency with an associated subaortic stenosis. (a) High velocity flow distal to the stenosis can be seen with colour flow imaging (b). IM = mitral insufficiency. Note abbreviations VG = left ventricle

insufficiency should lead to a more detailed examination so that any masked associations can be diagnosed, for example a coarctation of the aorta or a discrete subaortic stenosis (Fig. 10.18).

Stenotic or insufficient mitral valves may also be associated with other malformations such as ventricular septal defects (Fig. 10.19), or there may be components of a complex malformation. Cardiomyopathies, mitral malformation, univentricular hearts, left-outflow tract obstructions, and atrioventricular defects are always im-portant factors when determining the prognosis of a lesion detected prenatally.

The diagnosis of atrioventricular insufficiency helps in determining the postnatal course of malformations involving an atrioventricular valve anomaly/atrioventricular canal defects (Fig. 10.20), or univentricular hearts, or double outlet right ventricles with complete atrioventricular canal defects (Fig. 10.21), in which early surgical repair or cavopulmonary circulation is indicated after birth.

A single atrioventricular valve may be a mitral valve with tricuspid atresia, a tricuspid valve with a mitral atresia, a common atrioventricular valve in atrioventricular defect (Fig. 10.22). Whatever the defect, the assessment

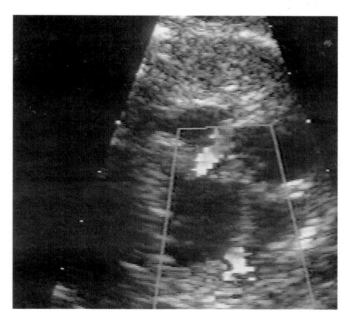

Fig. 10.19
In this example there is mitral insufficiency with a dilated left ventricle. There is an associated apical ventricular septal defect, which could easily be missed without the use of colour flow imaging

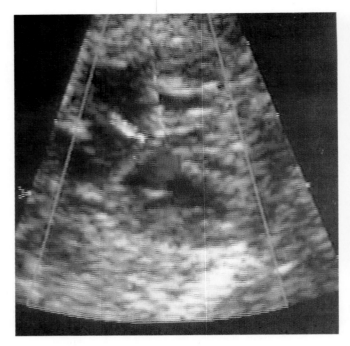

Fig. 10.20
An combined atrioventricular canal/valve defect. The finding of
A-V insufficiency in this condition helps determine the
prognosis for the fetus with this lesion in postnatal life.

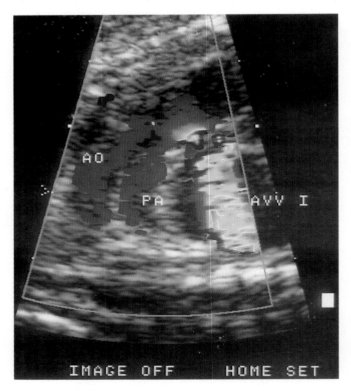

Fig. 10.21
Complete atrioventricular canal defect with a double outlet right
ventricle. The aorta and pulmonary artery are seen arising from
tha same ventricle.

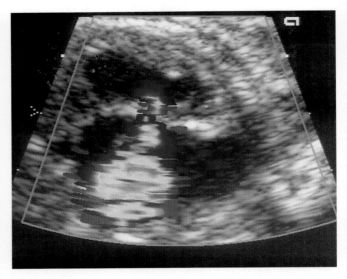

Fig. 10.22
A single atrioventricular valve may be a mitral in tricuspid
atresia, a tricuspid valve in mitral atresia, a common
atrioventricular valve in atrioventricular defect or 'cor
bilocular', as seen in this image. Whatever the precise defect,
the assessment of valvular function is important in trying to
predict the postnatal course and the type of palliative surgery
feasible. It is obvious that a precise diagnosis is valuable when
counselling the parents about the potential problems that lie
ahead

of valvular function is important in trying to predict the
postnatal course and the type of palliative surgery feasible. It is obvious that a precise diagnosis is important to
assist in counselling the parents about the potential problems that lie ahead.

THE PULMONIC AND AORTIC VALVES

Sigmoid valve insufficiencies are rare occurrences during
fetal life. An aortic insufficiency is rarely detected in the
presence of ventricular septal defects and could indicate
an infundibular localization or an aortic valve dysplasia.
More often, it leads to a possible diagnosis of truncus
arteriosus or valvular dysplasia and therefore points toward a
vascular anomaly. Diastolic flow below the aortic valves
leads to the diagnosis of an aortoventricular tunnel.

Significant pulmonary insufficiency is equally very rare.
At first, the diagnosis to consider is the syndrome of absent
pulmonary valves with or without a ventricular septal
defect. Ebstein's anomalies or dysplasias of the tricuspid
valves are detected by 2D echodoppler. Tricuspid insufficiency is usually easily detected by pulsed Doppler techniques, but determining the prognosis is based on the
anatomy of the valve, the size and function of the right
ventricle, and the function of the left ventricle. Pulmonary
functional anatomy must also be assessed to help in determining the prognosis. Where there is substantial tricus-

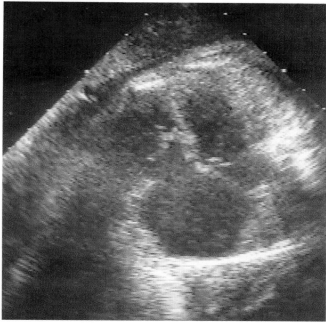

(a)

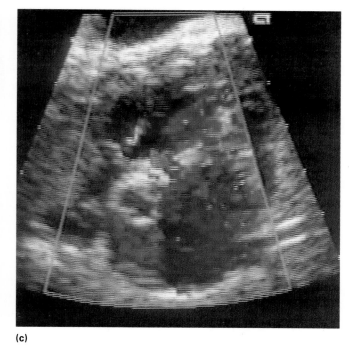

(c)

(b)

Fig. 10.23

Suspected pulmonary atresia. A real time image (a), with the suspected pulmonary atresia (b), and the demonstration of pulmonary insufficiency (c) with the aid of colour Doppler. This finding excludes the possibility of complete pulmonary atresia.

pid regurgitation, the pulmonary arterial dimensions may be very small without motion of the valves and reverse flow from the ductus arteriosus may be seen. Colour Doppler provides important information regarding the flow in the main pulmonary artery and the infundibulum of the right ventricle. If pulmonary insufficiency is detected, no matter how small, it excludes an associated pulmonary atresia (Fig. 10.23). The calculation of the tricuspid velocities and gradients are similarly important to determine if the right ventricular pressures are normal or raised. With this information it is possible to postulate on the most likely pulmonary haemodynamics that will occur after the neonatal changes in the pulmonary circulation.

When only one vessel and one annulus arising from the heart is visualized, the precise diagnosis is sometimes difficult to reach. The detection of a valvular leakage suggests the diagnosis of a truncus arteriosus rather than of a pulmonary atresia with ventricular septal defect.

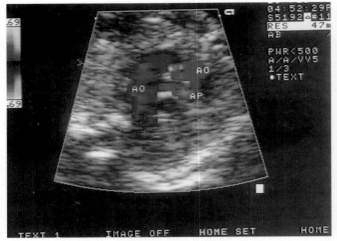

(a)

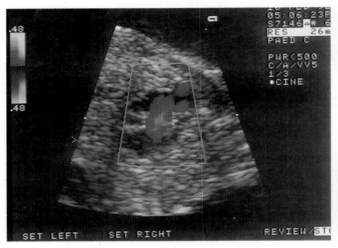

(b)

Fig. 10.24

The pulmonary haemodynamics are a major component of the prognosis of most of the right-sided obstructive lesions and of the conotruncal malformations. In this case antegrade flow through the dictus arteriosus can be demonstrated. Compare this with Fig. 10.25, where there is retrograde flow through the ductus.

Outlet obstruction

Pulmonary haemodynamics are a major component in assessing the prognosis of most of the right-sided obstructive lesions and of the conotruncal malformations. The size of the vessel, the direction of flow, the detection of a subpulmonary atresia or severe stenosis, and the aspect of the pulmonary bifurcation are all major factors in deciding the technique of neonatal surgery and it is therefore very important to assess all these parameters prenatally. Antegrade flow (Fig. 10.24) and retrograde flow (Fig. 10.25) through the ductus can be clearly demonstrated. The localization of the pulmonary artery can be equally well defined as well as its bifurcation and the vascularization

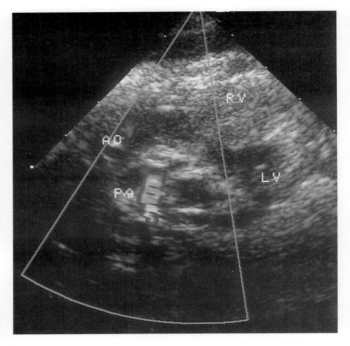

Fig. 10.25

Retrograde flow through the ductus arteriosus. This finding is important in the assessment of right sided heart lesions, compare with Fig. 10.24.

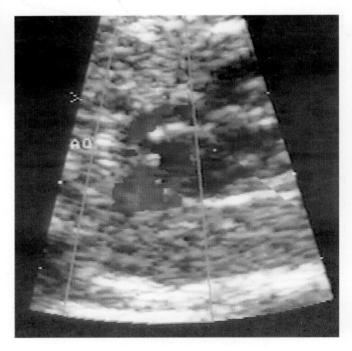

Fig. 10.26

Colour Doppler image of the diminutive but permeable ascending aorta overriding an infundibular ventricular septal defect in the case of interrupted aortic arch

of the right and left pulmonary arteries.

The aortic haemodynamic profile is similar to the pul-

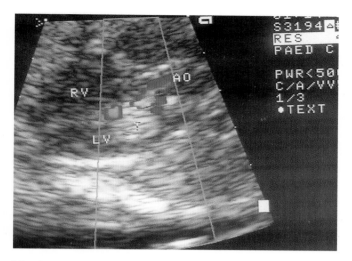

Fig. 10.27
The haemodynamic effect of a ventricular cardiac tumour can be assessed with CDI. In this case the tumour appears to be obstructing tha aortic outflow tract. Urgent neonatal surgery will be required to allow the heart to function after birth.

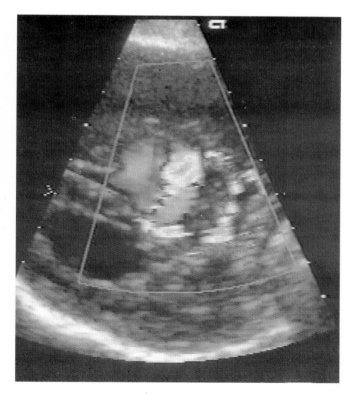

Fig. 10.28
The diagnosis of fistulae formation has been enhanced by colour Doppler. For instance, fistulae can be easily demonstrated in the liver or in the cerebral circulation

monary haemodynamic patterns. Retrograde flow from the ductus to the ascending aorta is demonstrated in hypoplastic left heart syndromes and this finding is especially useful in atypical forms of this condition. Colour Doppler brings

well-defined images of the diminutive but permeable ascending aorta overriding an infundibular ventricular septal defect in the case of interrupted aortic arch (Fig. 10.26).

Evaluation of the anatomy and function of the whole left outflow tract to detect anomalies at various levels is possible with the improved imaging allowed by colour Doppler. It is important to visualize the tract at the aortic root, at the aortic and mitral valvular levels, at the supravalvular and subvalvular levels, in addition to assessing left ventricular anatomy and function. Colour Doppler helps detect a partial restriction of the foramen ovale and/or tricuspid insufficiency, both important findings in hypoplastic left heart syndromes. Colour Doppler can also help detect mitral insufficiency or stenosis (or a combination of both) in the case of aortic stenosis or coarctations of the aorta.

Where ventricular septal defects are associated with aortic root anomalies, colour Doppler techniques improve the analysis of the anatomic anomaly, particularly of the subaortic outflow tract, which could be stenotic because of a membrane or a deviated subaortic canal muscle. This, in turn, could lead to further obstruction and is frequently a part of a more serious disease of the aortic arch. Colour Doppler is also useful in the detection of obstructive tumoral lesions below the aortic valves, thus helping to determine if urgent neonatal surgery is required (Fig. 10.27).

FISTULA FORMATION

The diagnosis of fistulae formation has been enhanced by the addition of colour Doppler to the cardiac examination. Fistulae are easy to demonstrate in the liver or in the cerebral circulation (Fig. 10.28). Other types are much more difficult to detect. In pulmonary atresia with an intact interventricular septum, the coronary fistula to the right ventricle will hinder complete repair after birth (Fig. 10.29), and is therefore important to diagnose/exclude.

CONCLUSION

When a complex congenital heart lesion has been diagnosed, an evaluation of all the anatomical and haemodynamic components is indicated to establish the fetal and, more importantly, the postnatal prognosis: a pulmonary arterial atresia or severe hypoplasia will interfere with the feasibility and long-term results of palliative surgery; an insufficiency of a common atrioventricular valve will increase if there is a need for an aortopulmonary shunt, with early deterioration of the valvular tissue and the high probability of early valvular replacement.

This overview of fetal cardiology supports the introduction of colour Doppler techniques in fetal cardiology by illustrating the major advances it brings to fetal/paediatric cardiology. All the flow patterns are assessed

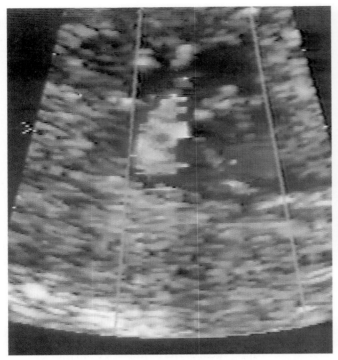

(a)

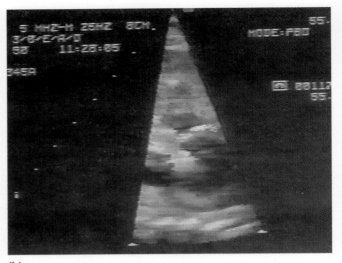

(b)

Fig. 10.29

Fistulae in the heart can be more difficult to diagnose. In this case of pulmonary atresia with an intact interventricular septum (a), the coronary fistula to the right ventricle (b) will hinder proper surgery after birth. Consequently, it is important to diagnose or exclude these associations if possible antenatally.

step by step using colour Doppler studies combined with con-
tinuous and pulsed wave examinations. In the fetus, this is currently the best technique capable of providing such important information about the fetal haemodynamic status, and about the natural history of congenital heart dis-eases before and after birth. Colour Doppler flow mapping improves our prenatal diagnostic capability, providing valuable information that will help in determining prognosis/surgical outcome. In this respect it has been the most important breakthrough in the field of fetal echo-cardiography in recent years.

CHAPTER 11

New horizons in Doppler imaging

Stuart Campbell, Kevin Harrington and Colin Deane

INTRODUCTION

Stuart Campbell

The last 10 years have seen a rapid development in Doppler technology, such that state of the art machines can now incorporate colour/pulsed Doppler while retaining the ability to produce first class B-mode images. These improvements have expanded the possible applications for Doppler ultrasound. This book is in itself testament to the potential for such technology in obstetrics and maternal-fetal medicine. There is no doubt that in the next few years new applications of existing machinery, and innovative technology will continue to expand the horizons for Doppler and blood flow imaging.

This chapter is a combination of short presentations on some of the new applications that are likely to gain prominence in the coming years.

MEASUREMENT OF VOLUME FLOW WITH CVI-Q

Kevin Harrington

Doppler ultrasound provides indirect information about blood flow changes, mainly through measurement of resistance indices and velocities. This knowledge is used in many areas of medicine, providing valuable data that helps in the clinical management of patients. Actual changes in volume flow (Q, calculated from the product of time averaged mean velocity and the cross-sectional area of the vessel lumen) would be the ideal in many circumstances, but current methods of measuring volume flow using real-time and Doppler ultrasound are limited by the large degree of error that occurs with these calculations.

1 The main sources of error are measurement of the vessel diameter, especially if the vessel is of small calibre, and in the calculations of velocities.
2 Even though the sources of error can be minimized and variations in measurement kept to a minimum in a controlled setting.
3 Estimates of volume flow based on B-mode/Doppler data are not routinely used in the clinical setting.

A new technique, which has the potential to provide information on actual changes in the volume of flow, is now available. This system uses M-mode to measure the time-varying vessel diameter, and colour

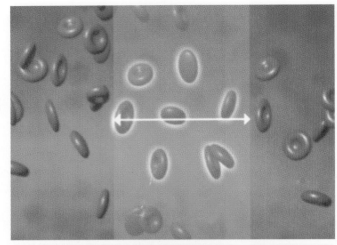
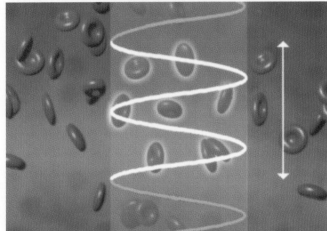
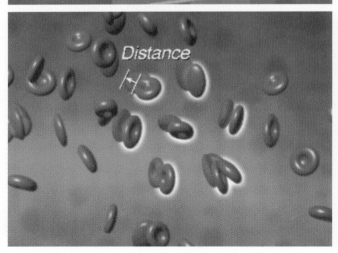

Fig. 11.1
A diagrammatic representation of the principle utilized in time domain processing. The movement of a packet of signals can be tracked in time, and the distance travelled by the signals measured by cross correlation. The velocity component can now be calculated. Colour velocity imaging utilizes this information to produce a colour map of changing velocities in the ultrasound beam.

velocity imaging, which differs from Doppler in that it calculates positional change (rather than frequency shift), to measure velocities.

Colour velocity imaging

Colour velocity imaging (CVI) measures flow velocity within vessels using time of flight changes between consecutive pulses. The ultrasound wave identifies 'packets' of signals, e.g. from some blood cells, that have a distinctive reflected signature. A second wave identifies the new position of the same packet of signals a short time later. The distance travelled by the packet of cells can be calculated over time, independent of the frequency of the ultrasound signal. Up to 20 million of these calculations can be performed every second, and this information is utilized to calculate the velocity shift (Fig. 11.1).

The proposed advantage of this approach, when compared with Doppler, is that the use of shorter pulse lengths allows better resolution of the velocity profile, and the technique is less susceptible to the limitations of aliasing (Fig. 11.2). The real advantage of this more precise quantification of velocity shift is in its potential to fulfil part of the equation for volume flow. Combined with M-mode which provides a reliable continuous measurement of vessel diameter, it is now possible with ultrasound to accurately measure volume flow within a vessel in a clinical setting (CVI-Q).

Calculation of volume flow with CVI-Q

CVI-Q, therefore, combines CVI technology with M-mode imaging of a vessel to assess vessel diameter and velocity shift instantaneously. The shorter pulse length required for CVI means that a minimum of

velocity information is lost in transmission time, when compared with Doppler. The first step in obtaining CVI-Q measurements is a clear colour velocity image, with an angle of insonation greater than 30° and less than 70°. It is important that the transducer lies longitudinal to, and in the middle of, the vessel. By moving the transducer across the vessel it is possible to ensure that the middle of the vessel is being insonated. In duplex mode, the CVI-Q image appears as an M-mode image with superimposed colour. It is possible to check if you remain in the midline by observing the range of colour in the image, and by ensuring that the amount of dias-tolic flow is appropriate for the vessel being examined (Fig. 11.3).

The criteria for obtaining reliable measurement of volume flow with CVI-Q are shown below. When compared with Doppler there is a greater emphasis on obtaining an accurate measurement of the angle of insonation of the vessel, and being in the exact centre of the vessel at the time of the examination.

- Straight portion of vessel (no curvature or turbulence);
- Vessel >3 mm diameter;
- Angle >30<70°;
- Optimum colour signal;
- Centre of vessel (no tapering);
- Accurate measurement of angle of insonation;
- Satisfactory velocity and flow patterns.

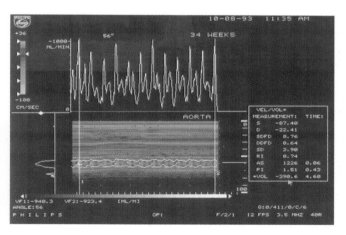

Fig. 11.3
CVI-Q image obtained from the fetal aorta of a healthy fetus and the same vessel in a fetus suffering the effects of anaemia. CVI-Q combines the information derived from CVI, with the information derived from a simultaneous M-mode signal, to create a measurement of the actual flow within a vessel. This has the advantage over Doppler of measuring changes in volume rather than resistance/velocity, which do not always reflect the precise changes in the supply through a particular vessel or organ. Because of the greater operator dependance with CVI-Q in its present form, it is likely to complement rather than replace Doppler ultrasound.

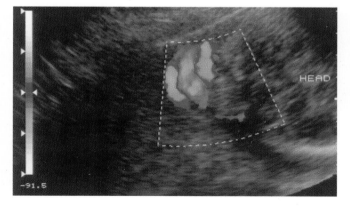

Fig. 11.2
Colour velocity image of the umbilical cord encircling the fetal head. The advantage of velocity imaging, when compared with Doppler, is that the use of shorter pulse lengths allows better resolution of the velocity profile and the technique does not suffer less from the limitations of aliasing.

It is very important to ensure that the angle is correct before proceeding with calculations. A velocity profile and a volume flow profile are presented on screen. This is the final checkpoint that allows you to ensure that the vessel was being insonated at the midline.

In-vitro studies

Using a hand held 5 MHz linear transducer in a flow rig we measured flow at different rates and angles. For flow rates ≥ 40 ml/min accuracy of flow was well within 10%, within a range of angles from 30–70°. At angles above this, velocity errors made quantitative measurement of flow unreliable. At angles below 30°, the increased error in calculating vessel diameter led to large errors of area estimation, and hence made flow measurements unreliable.

Potential applications for CVI-Q

Initial studies suggest that measurement of volume flow with CVI-Q provides reliable data that reflects the actual volume of flow within a vessel, with acceptable variability. Any disease or therapeutic process that is characterized by a change in volume flow is ideal for CVI-Q studies; investigation of vascular disease, in surgical work, the results of the operation might be monitored more carefully; the effect of drug therapy on vessels and organs may be assessed more accurately. These are simply a few initial ideas. No doubt the reader will already have thought of a potential use in his or her chosen area of expertise.

CVI-Q requires different working practices compared to the use of colour/pulsed Doppler. There are different limitations with each technique. There are stricter criteria for producing accurate measurements of volume flow with CVI-Q, when compared with Doppler. CVI-Q is more time-consuming. It is likely, therefore, to complement rather than replace Doppler ultrasound, providing more accurate and valuable data where Doppler investigations are known to be unreliable, or where changes in volume rather than resistance is the most important feature of a condition. Ongoing CVI-Q studies will ultimately determine the most useful role for this technology in medical practice.

THREE-DIMENSIONAL COLOUR FLOW ULTRASOUND

Colin Deane

Conventional colour flow imaging (colour Doppler and colour velocity imaging) uses a similar format to B-mode images, providing flow information in a 2-D slice

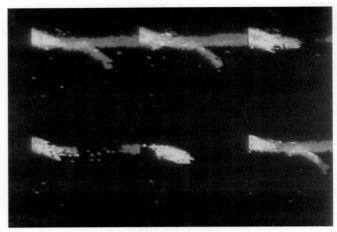

(a)

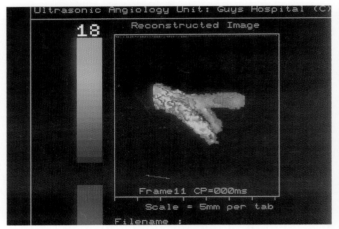

(b)

Fig. 11.4
With three-dimensional imaging a series of colour flow 'slices' are recorded as the transducer moves across the axis of the vessel (a). The imge is reconstructed as a surface image of the vessel and is viewed obliquely (b).

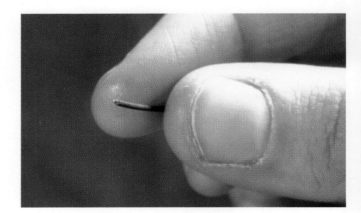

Fig. 11.5
A 20 MHz pulsed Doppler catheter. The catheter is 4F with a tip diameter of 1mm. The transducer is annular in shape with a lumen to permit insertion of a guide wire.

in the axis of the transducer. The colour 'map' changes in real time with a frame rate dependent on the area scanned, the colour line density, the number of pulses per line used and the pulse repetition frequency. In the sense that flow changes with time.

There are, however, alternative ways in which acquired B-mode and flow data can be displayed.[4] There has been recent interest in providing flow images in three spatial dimensions (so-called 3-D), for example by providing 'solid' images of flow signals in a vessel.

The difficulties of 3-D ultrasound are twofold: acquisition of data is complex and display of a 3-D image in two dimensions is a compromise. Acquisition can be achieved in real time by use of 2-D arrays (although to date this has not been applied to flow imaging),[5] or over a period of time using a conventional transducer and moving it in the third plane to provide a series of slices, which are stored and used to reconstruct an image. For reconstructions of flow imaging, data acquisition must be made over a least one cardiac cycle if dynamic representations are to be made This can be time-consuming.

The processed data can be displayed as the surface of the colour flow image which can then be viewed from different directions (Fig. 11.4). Sections of the image can be removed so as to view the flow signals in the plane of choice.

Perceived advantages of true 3-D flow imaging are that vascular anatomy may be displayed more clearly, that flow measurements may be more accurately made and that 3-D velocity vectors within vessels may be measured.

INTRAVASCULAR DOPPLER ULTRASOUND

Colin Deane

Intravascular Doppler ultrasound catheters are commercially available for velocity imaging within vessels. The advantage of these invasive catheters is that high frequency ultrasound (typically 20 MHz) can be used because of the absence of intervening tissue. Consequently, they are sensitive to low flow velocities. The small size of Doppler catheters (Fig. 11.5) allows them to be mounted in conjunction with pressure transducers or in combination with interventional catheters. The accuracy of measurements is highly dependent on the catheter's position within the lumen, careful placement is necessary to ensure the sample volume of the Doppler transducer is within the desired area of interest. Applications to date have mainly been in the study of adult coronary flows.

COLOUR FLOW IMAGING — AMPLITUDE/POWER DISPLAYS

Colin Deane

Recently, some ultrasound manufacturers have introduced amplitude displays as an alternative means of showing colour-coded flow information. Already there are several terms used to describe the displays including power Doppler, Doppler energy and ultrasound angiology.

Colour Doppler signal processing techniques provide an estimate of the mean frequency (and its variance) and the amplitude of the signal within the selected sample volume (Fig. 11.6 a to c). Traditionally, displays have been based on the direction and magnitude of frequency shifts, for instance by using different hues or saturations of blue and red. Since the flow velocities in arteries vary throughout the cardiac cycle, a changing colour image will be displayed, dependent on the flow waveform and the frame rate of the image.

The amplitude of the flow signal, however, has less variation throughout the cardiac cycle because it is dependent on the number of reflectors rather than their velocity. Colour maps based solely on the amplitude of the Doppler signal can, therefore, use frame averaging techniques to boost the signal to noise ratio at the

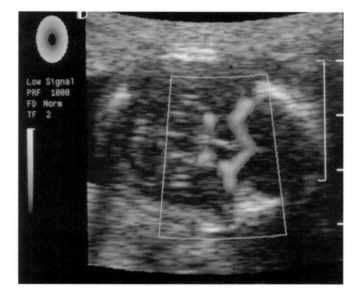

Fig. 11.7
Amplitude map of a fetal circle of Willis. Directional information has been sacrificed in order to gain better sensitivity to low flow velocities. (Image courtesy of Diasonics.)

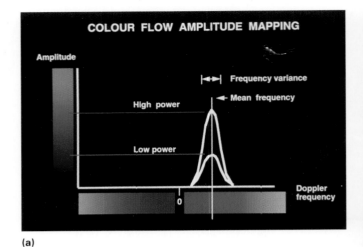

(a)

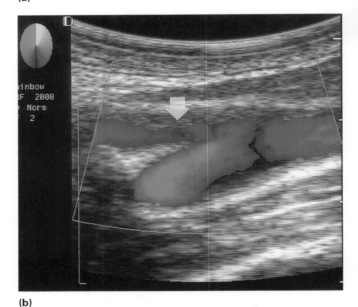

(b)

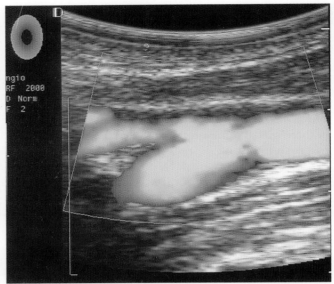

(c)

Fig. 11.6

(a) Colour flow imaging signal processing provides an estimate of mean frequency, frequency variance and the amplitude (or power) of the signal. The diagram shows two signals of the same mean frequency (as shown on the blue/red colour bar). If an amplitude display is used, the high power signal can be allocated a different hue from the low power signal (as shown on the amber bar). Conversely, signals of the same power will be allocated the same amplitude signal regardless of mean frequency. (b) A bifurcation imaged with a conventional colour scale based on a frequency shift. The ultrasound beam/flow vectors produce positive and negative shifts in the vessel and some regions of the vessel contain no colour image because of poor beam/flow angles (arrow). (c) The same bifurcation imaged with an amplitude map at the same pulse repetition frequency as in (b) The colour is more uniform and there is better filling of the vessel. Note the change in hue near the edge of the flow.

expense of a dynamic image. In addition, the amplitude estimate of the signal is less noisy than the frequency estimate. As a result, amplitude displays are claimed to be more sensitive to low flow velocities than frequency/velocity maps.

The characteristics of amplitude maps – high sensitivity, low temporal resolution and (if amplitude alone is used) loss of directional information – produce images that are complementary to conventional colour and spectral images. The maps are used best to detect the presence of flow and provide an assessment of perfusion in the scan plane (Fig. 11.7).

Because the colour signal in a sample volume is dependent on the amount of scatterers, small vessels of a diameter lower than the sample volume size will produce a low amplitude reflection (Fig. 11.8). Similarly, at the edge of larger vessels, amplitude is reduced in sample volumes which include the vessel wall. If a graded

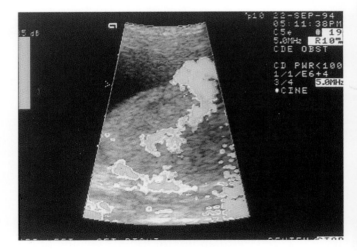

Fig. 11.8

Colour Doppler image of placental perfusion using a colour amplitude display (colour Doppler energy).

amplitude map is used, these reduced amplitudes appear as a different colour from high amplitude regions (Fig. 11.6c).

One notable artifact that amplitude maps can suffer from is caused by depth dependent attenuation of ultrasound. The reduction in signal amplitude thus caused may result in changes in map hues or saturations.

REFERENCES

1 Eik-Nes SH, Brubakk AO, Ulstein MK. (1980) Measurement of human fetal blood flow. *Br Med J* **280**: 283–6.

2 Griffin D, Cohen-Overbeek T, Campbell S. (1993) Fetal and uteroplacental blood flow. *Clin Obstet Gynaecol* **10**: 565–602.

3 Gill RW. (1985) Measurement of blood flow by ultrasound: Accuracy and sources of error. *Ultrasound Med Biol* **11**: 625–31.

4 Beach KW. Three-dimensional ultrasound imaging of arteries. In: *Diagnostic Vascular Ultrasound*. Edited by Laos KH. London: Edward Arnold, 1992.

5 Smith SW, Trahey GE, von-Ramm OTAD. (1992) Two-dimensional arrays for medical ultrasound. *Ultrason-Imaging* **14**: 213–33.

Normal ranges for commonly used Doppler indices of the uteroplacental and fetal circulation

R. G. Carpenter and Kevin Harrington
Charts prepared by Dr. R. G. Carpenter

Uterine artery resistance index (RI)

Resistance in the uterine circulation falls during pregnancy. An elevated RI in the second half of pregnancy is associated with increased morbidity, as a consequence of pre-eclampsia, intrauterine growth retardation, and placental abruption in particular. The addition of the presence of early diastolic notching of the flow velocity waveform as the definition of an abnormal waveform results in a high sensitivity and positive predictive value (see Chapter 4).

Umbilical artery pulsatility index (PI)

End diastolic frequencies are usually present on the umbilical artery waveform from about 16 weeks. The pulsatility index continues to fall throughout pregnancy. High resistance in the umbilical arterial circulation in the second half of pregnancy suggests a failure of placental development. It may be useful in determining the aetiology of fetal smallness.

Middle cerebral pulsatility index (PI)

Resistance in the cerebral circulation tends to gradually fall in the second half of pregnancy, probably secondary to the changes in the partial pressures of oxygen and carbon dioxide. An exaggerated drop in the middle cerebral artery (MCA) PI (<5th centile) suggests hypoxaemia. Where there is a change in the growth velocity of a fetus, a fall in the MCA PI may be the first sign of uteroplacental insufficiency.

Middle cerebral time averaged mean velocity (TAV)

There is a rise in the middle cerebral artery time averaged velocity (TAV) in conjunction with the fall in the MCA PI. An unusually high MCA TAV suggests hypoxaemia (+ low MCA PI) or anaemia (normal MCA PI).

Thoracic aorta pulsatility index (PI)

Resistance in the thoracic aorta (TA) remains relatively constant in the second half of pregnancy (compare with the umbilical artery PI), reflecting steady state cardiac/arterial haemodynamics. A rise in the TA PI, and in particular loss of end diastolic frequencies in the thoracic aorta, are associated with the development of fetal acidaemia. These changes usually occur after changes in the cerebral circulation, and may occur independently of changes in the umbilical arterial circulation.

Thoracic aorta time averaged mean velocity (TAV)

There is a rise in time averaged velocity (TAV) in the aorta until approximately 32 weeks, when velocities appear to plateau. Low velocities in the aorta suggests acidaemia, especially if they occur alongside a rise in aortic resistance. High velocities in the aorta suggest anaemia.

Umbilical artery/middle cerebral artery PI ratio

In the preterm hypoxaemic growth retarded fetus resistance in the umbilical arteries rises, whereas resistance falls in the middle cerebral arteries. A ratio of these two values may be helpful in the early detection of the growth retarded fetus. A high value suggests hypoxaemia secondary to uteroplacental insufficiency.

Middle cerebral artery/thoracic aorta PI ratio

Reduced MCA resistance (low PI) suggests hypoxaemia, and increased aortic resistance (high PI) indicates the presence of fetal acidaemia. Changes occurring in these vessels can be highlighted by combining these two values as a ratio. The higher the value the greater the likelihood that the fetus is hypoxic and acidaemic.

Middle cerebral artery PI x thoracic aorta TAV

Changes in cerebral resistance (low MCA PI) can be highlighted if multiplied by aortic velocities. A low value suggests that cerebral and systemic changes to the cardiovascular system are necessary to maintain cerebral oxygenation.

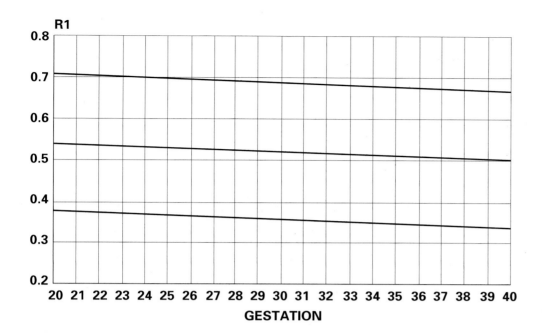

Fig. App. 1
Uterine artery resistance
index (RI) 5/95th centile

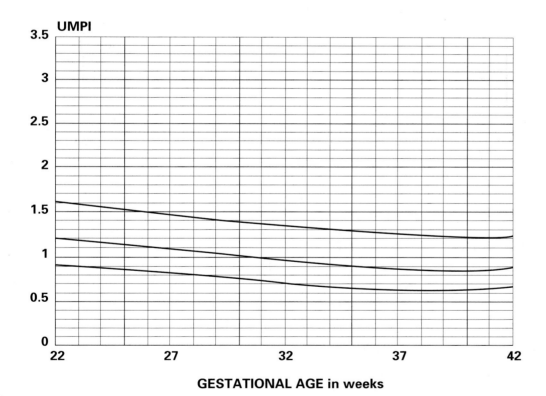

Fig. App. 2
Umbilical artery
pulsatility index (PI)

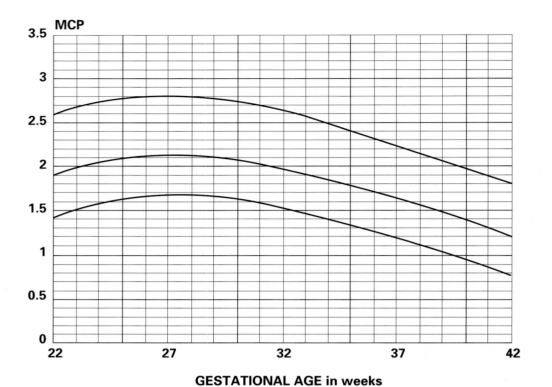

Fig. App. 3
Middle cerebral pulsatility index (PI)

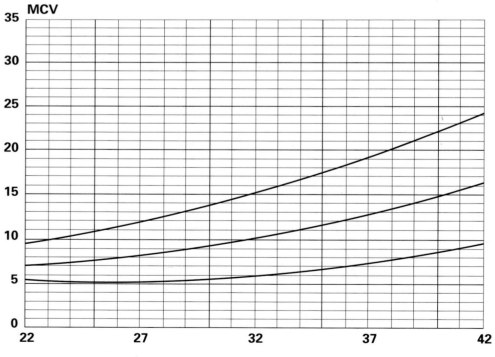

Fig. App. 4
Middle cerebral time averaged mean velocity (TAV)

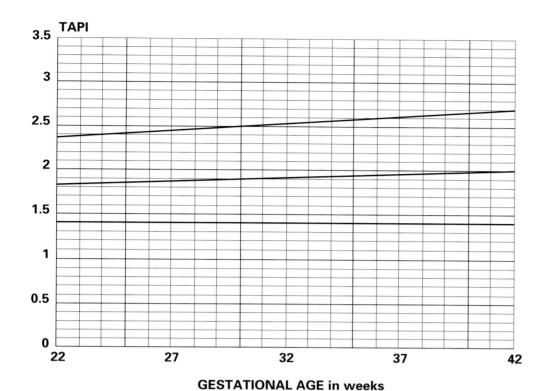

Fig. App. 5
Thoracic aorta pulsatility
index (PI)

GESTATIONAL AGE in weeks

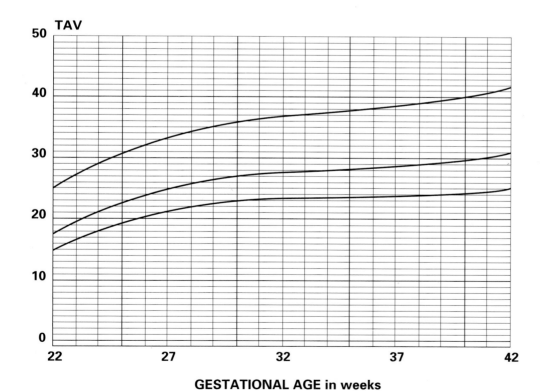

Fig. App. 6
Thoracic aorta time
averaged mean velocity
(TAV)

GESTATIONAL AGE in weeks

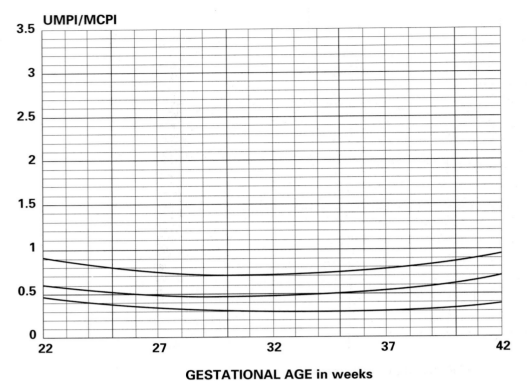

GESTATIONAL AGE in weeks

Fig. App. 7
Umbilical artery/middle
cerebral artery PI ratio

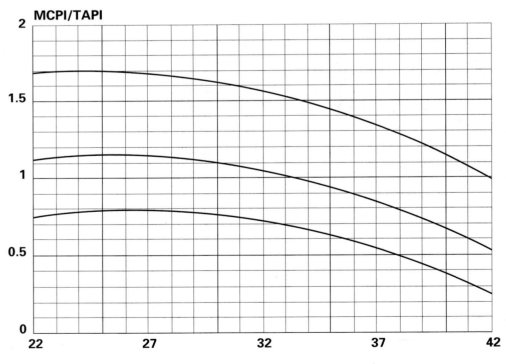

GESTATIONAL AGE in weeks

Fig. App. 8
Middle cerebral
artery/thoracic aorta PI
ratio

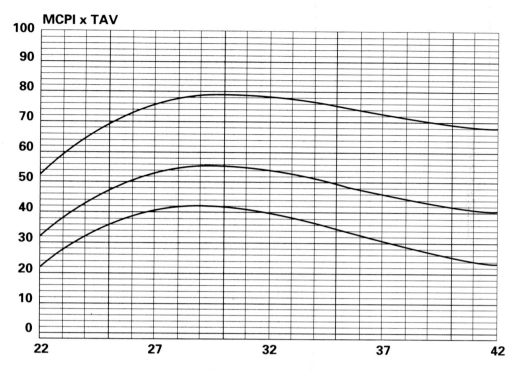

Fig. App. 9
Middle cerebral artery
PI x thoracic aorta TAV

GESTATIONAL AGE in weeks

Index